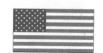

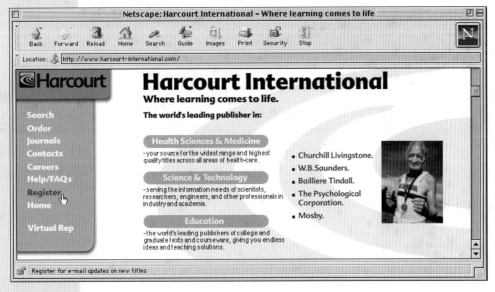
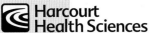

COLOR ATLAS OF BURN CARE

WB SAUNDERS
An imprint of Harcourt Publishers Limited

© Harcourt Publishers Limited 2001

 is a registered trademark of Harcourt Publishers Limited

The right of Juan P. Barret, MD and David N. Herndon, MD to be identified as authors of this work has been asserted by them in accordance with the Copyright, Designs and Patents Act 1988

First published 2001

ISBN   0 7020 25089

British Library Cataloguing in Publication Data
A catalogue record for this book is available from the British Library

Library of Congress Cataloging in Publication Data
A catalog record for this book is available from the Library of Congress

Note
Medical knowledge is constantly changing. As new information becomes available, changes in treatment, procedures, equipment and the use of drugs become necessary. The authors, contributors and the publishers have taken care to ensure that the information given in this text is accurate and up to date. However, readers are strongly advised to confirm that the information, especially with regard to drug usage, complies with the latest legislation and standards of practice.

Printed in China

Commissioning Editor: Serena Bureau
Project Manager: Helen Sofio
Designer: Greg Smith

The
Publisher's
Policy is to use
paper manufactured
from sustainable forests

COLOR ATLAS OF BURN CARE

JUAN P. BARRET, MD
Burns and Plastic Surgeon
Department of Plastic Surgery
University Hospital Groningen
Groningen
The Netherlands

DAVID N. HERNDON, MD
Chief of Staff, Shriners Burns Hospital
Jesse H. Jones Distinguished Chair in Burn Surgery
Professor of Surgery and Pediatrics
Department of Surgery
University of Texas Medical Branch
Galveston, Texas
USA

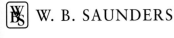 W. B. SAUNDERS

LONDON EDINBURGH NEW YORK PHILADELPHIA ST LOUIS SYDNEY TORONTO 2001

INTRODUCTION TO BURN CARE

Juan P. Barret, MD and David N. Herndon, MD

There have been many improvements in the treatment of burn patients over the past few decades. Over 50 years ago we learned the importance of burn resuscitation, and the impact that delay in resuscitation had on burn mortality. It was clear after a while that, despite our efforts on resuscitation, burn patients succumbed to burn wound infection. Control of infection was the second revolution that occurred in burn care. In the late 1960s and early 1970s new topical antimicrobial agents became available. Those new agents, along with the beginning of the new era of burn excision and grafting, were grounds for the birth of modern burn care. Skin banks, early excision and grafting, and new skin substitutes came soon afterwards. During the 1980s there was a consolidation of early excision and closure of the burn wound, which, nowadays, is the current standard of care for full thickness burns. Extensive programs of early closure of burn wounds, along with topical antimicrobial agents, have made the occurrence of burn wound sepsis extremely rare. Also, a better understanding of the pathophysiology of the burn syndrome has lead to the modulation of the catabolic response. Recombinant human growth factors, such as human growth hormone and insulin-like growth factor, and other new drugs such as oxandrolone, have been proved to have an important effect in the modulation of catabolism after burn trauma. The advent of high-frequency ventilation and new methods of conventional ventilation have improved survival after inhalation injury, but, despite all our efforts, respiratory distress syndrome is still the most common cause of death among burn patients. New areas for improvement and research are the development of new skin substitutes, better means for delivery of new growth factors, and new drug therapies for inhalation injury. Tissue engineering, gene therapy with growth factors, and gas exchange membranes, among others, will be the new achievements of the next millennium.

The former improvements in burn care have led to improvements in day-to-day patient care. Nowadays, the plan of patient care starts before the patient is admitted. As soon as the burn team is aware of the situation, a master plan is outlined. All disciplines are involved, so that a discharge plan is started that will be revised as the patient improves and progresses. 'State of the art' techniques of nursing, surgery, rehabilitation, etc., are implemented, so that the best possible outcome is obtained. When summarized in figures, we can state that currently all pediatric and young adult burn patients, regardless of the extent of their injuries, should be considered candidates for survival. Many reports from institutions throughout the world support this statement. To speak for all the others, the burn size that kills 50% of patients (LD_{50}) among pediatric burn victims at the Shriners Burns Hospital (SBH), Galveston, Texas, is currently over 90% total body surface burned area. Similarly, in young adults, the LD_{50} at the Vall d'Hebron Hospital Burn Center in Barcelona, Spain is also over 90% total body surface burned area. There is also hope for our older burn patients. The LD_{50} at the latter institution among patients over 60 years old is 41% total body surface burned area.

The present atlas, intended as a quick reference and companion to *Total Burn Care*, compiles in a single issue a summary of the current treatment of burns at the SBH and at the University of Texas Medical Branch (UTMB) in Galveston that have led to these achievements. The contribution of experts from different countries makes it an extremely elaborated edition. The knowledge and insight provided by Dr David N. Herndon, Chief of Burns Services at SBH and UTMB, is combined with the expertise of Dr Juan P. Barret and Mr Peter Dziewulski (once burn surgeons in Galveston); together, these contributors have collated their experience and ideas, from Galveston, Texas, from Barcelona, Spain, and from London, UK. The disciplines of General Surgery and Plastic Surgery are united in a team of collegian surgeons in Galveston, at the bedside, and in the preparation of this *Color Atlas of Burn Care*. We hope that the reader will find this comprehensive approach to all practical issues of burn care useful, and that it will serve as a quick reference for day-to-day care.

With all our respect and dedication to burn victims.

September 1999

Groningen, The Netherlands and Galveston, Texas

DEDICATION

To our wives, Esther and Rose. Without them, none of this would
have been possible.

ACKNOWLEDGEMENTS

The authors would like to acknowledge Tina Garcia, Lewis Milutin,
and Sandy Baxter, from the Department of Graphic Services, for
their help in the preparation of the photographic material; Lucy
Behrends, Director of Medical Records, for her help with data
acquisition; and the Medical Staff Office administrative personnel,
for their support and day-to-day work.

CONTENTS

LIST OF CONTRIBUTORS

Juan P. Barret, MD
Burns and Plastic Surgeon
Department of Plastic Surgery
University Hospital Groningen
Groningen
The Netherlands
Formerly: Shriners Burns Hospital, University of Texas Medical
Branch, Galveston, Texas, USA, and
Hospital General 'Vall d'Hebron', Barcelona, Spain

Anthony N. Dardano, DO
Chief Resident in Plastic and Reconstructive Surgery
Department of Surgery
Division of Plastic Surgery
Shriners Burns Hospital
University of Texas Medical Branch
Galveston, Texas
USA

Peter Dziewulski, FRCS, FRCS (Plast)
Consultant Plastic Surgeon
St Andrews Centre for Plastic Surgery and Burns
Broomfield Hospital
Broomfield, Chelmsford, Essex
UK

John P. Heggers, PhD, FAAM, CWS
Director, Clinical Microbiology
Professor of Surgery (Plastic), Microbiology and Immunology
Division of Plastic Surgery
Shriners Burns Hospital
University of Texas Medical Branch
Galveston, Texas
USA

David N. Herndon, MD
Chief of Staff, Shriners Burns Hospital
Jesse H. Jones Distinguished Chair in Burn Surgery
Professor of Surgery and Pediatrics
Department of Surgery
Shriners Burns Hospital
University of Texas Medical Branch
Galveston, Texas
USA

Marc G. Jeschke, MD, MMS
Department of Surgery
Klinikum der Universität Regensburg
Klinikum und Poliklinik für Chirurgie Regensburg
Germany
Formerly: Research Fellow, Shriners Burns Hospital, Galveston,
Texas, USA

Ronald P. Mlcak, BA, RRT
Director of Respiratory Care
Department of Respiratory Care
Shriners Burns Hospital
University of Texas Medical Branch
Galveston, Texas
USA

Ray J. Nichols Jr, MD
Professor of Anesthesia
Chief of Anesthesiology
Shriners Burns Hospital for Children
University of Texas Medical Branch
Galveston, Texas
USA

Lynn A. 'Pete' Peterson, CRNA, MSN
Chief Nurse Anesthetist
Department of Anesthesia
Shriners Burns Hospital for Children
University of Texas Medical Branch
Galveston, Texas
USA

CHAPTER 1
THE BURN WOUND

Juan P. Barret, MD and Peter Dziewulski, FRCS, FRCS (Plast)

PATHOPHYSIOLOGY OF THE BURN WOUND

Types of Injuries and Clinical Examples

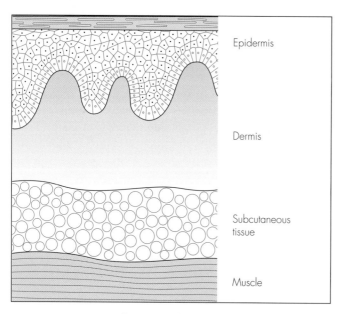

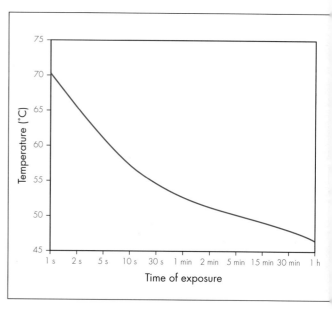

1.1.1.1 Diagram of normal skin. Note the architecture of the epidermal papillae and dermal crest. Their indentation is responsible for many physical properties of skin. Sweat glands and hair follicles are present deep in the dermal and subcutaneous tissue, and are responsible for re-epithelization of second-degree burns and donor sites.

1.1.1.2 Skin surface temperature needed to produce full thickness damage versus time. Adapted from Moritz AR and Heriques FC. AM J. Pathol 1947; 23: 695–720.

First Degree Burn

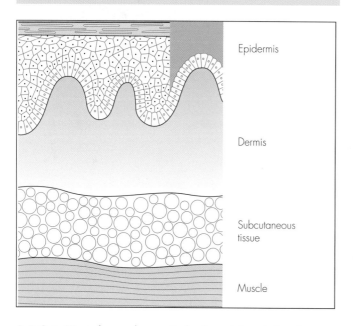

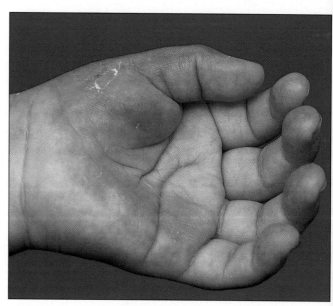

1.1.2.1 First-degree burn. Only the epidermis has been damaged.

1.1.2.2 First-degree burn to the palmar surface of an infant's hand. Note the red, hyperemic appearance of the surface, which, along with the hypersensibility and discomfort, is typical of these injuries.

Second Degree Burns (Partial Thickness)

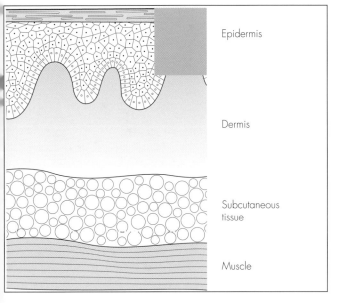

Epidermis

Dermis

Subcutaneous
tissue

Muscle

1.1.3.1 Superficial second-degree burn (superficial partial thickness). Epidermis and superficial (papillary) dermis have been damaged. Regeneration occurs by proliferation of epithelial cells from hair follicles and sweat gland ducts. Conversion to full thickness burns is rare, provided proper wound care is instituted.

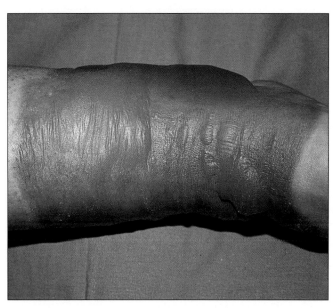

1.1.3.2 Superficial second-degree burn to the lower leg and forefoot. Blistering and extreme pain are typical of such injuries. Sensation is preserved with different degrees of hyperesthesia.

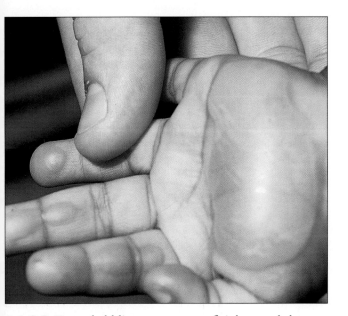

1.1.3.3 Extended blisters on a superficial second-degree contact burn to the palm of an infant.

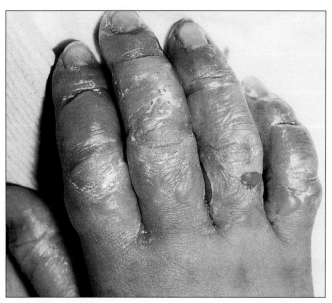

1.1.3.4 Superficial second-degree burns to the dorsa of the fingers. Splinting and early mobilization are important for treatment of burns in this location.

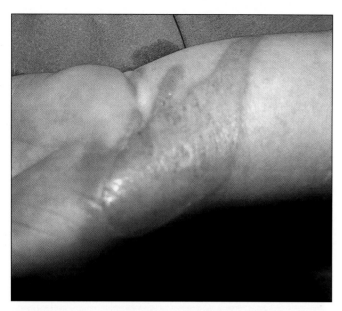

1.1.3.5 Typical appearance of superficial second-degree burns after removal of the blister. A moist, pink appearance that blanches with pressure, along with extreme pain and hyperesthesia, is common among these injuries.

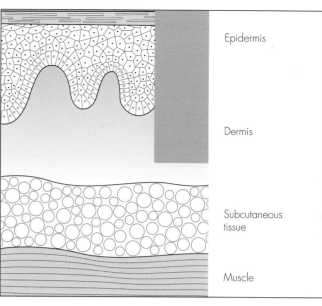

1.1.4.1 Deep second-degree burn (deep partial thickness burn). Epidermis, papillary dermis, and various depths of reticular (deep) dermis have been damaged. Regeneration occurs by proliferation of epithelial cells from hair follicles and sweat gland ducts. Concentration of such structures is less than in depths of superficial second-degree burns, and regeneration progresses more slowly Conversion to full thickness injury is possible.

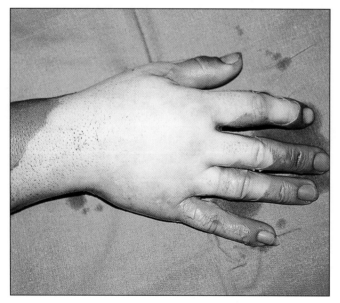

1.1.4.2 Deep second-degree burn to the dorsum of the hand. Note the pink-white appearance. These injuries tend to be hypoesthetic, presenting with less pain than superficial second-degree burns. Blistering does not normally occur, or is present many hours after the injury. A dry appearance is common.

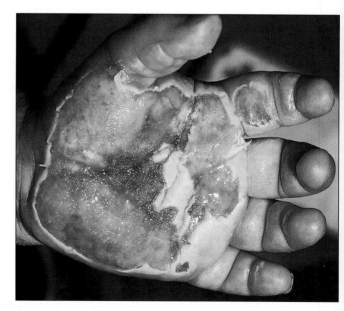

1.1.4.3 Deep second-degree burn to the palm. These injuries are best treated conservatively, and sequelae are rare.

Third Degree Burns (Full Thickness)

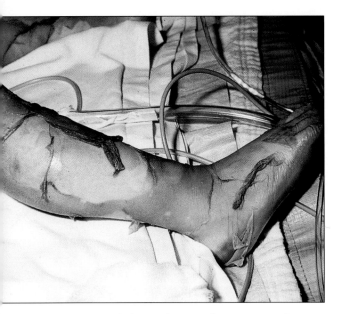

1.1.4.4 Deep second-degree burn to lower extremity.

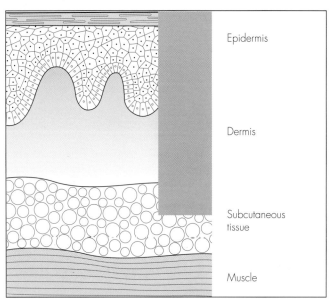

1.1.5.1 Third-degree burn (full thickness burn). Epidermis, papillary and reticular dermis, and different depths of subcutaneous tissue have been damaged. These injuries can not heal spontaneously, and treatment involves excision of all injured tissue.

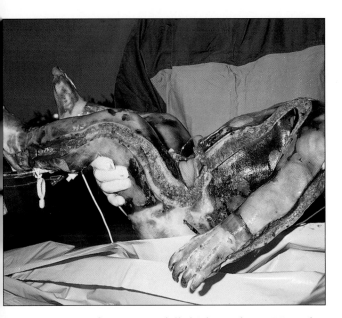

1.1.5.2 Ninety-five percent full thickness burn. Note the charred appearance.

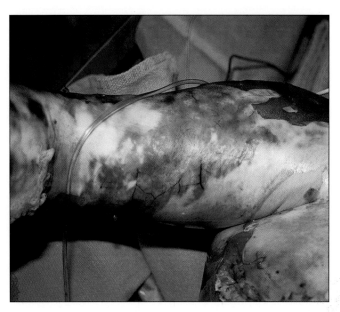

1.1.5.3 Third-degree burn to upper extremity. Note the thrombosed subcutaneous vascular plexus. Pain involved in these injuries is very low (usually with marginal partial thickness burns) or absent. All sensory terminations to the skin have been destroyed. The potential for infection if left nonexcised is very high.

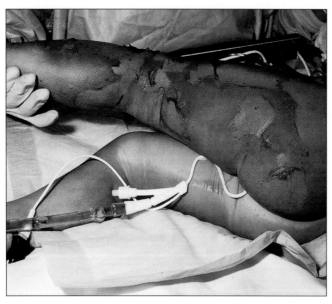

1.1.5.4 Third-degree burns to lower extremities. Flame injuries with differing degrees of carbon monoxide intoxication render a reddish appearance that can lead to confusion with that of partial thickness burns. Anesthesia and dry presentation, along with a red color that does not blanch with pressure, allow these injuries to be distinguished.

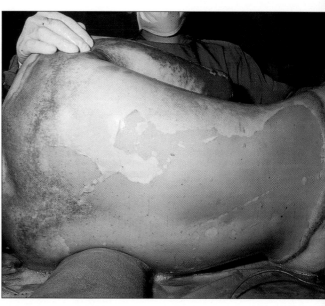

1.1.5.5 Third-degree burns to the back. The dry leather type appearance is typical of full thickness burns. Note that the periphery presents with deep partial thickness burns.

Fourth Degree Burns

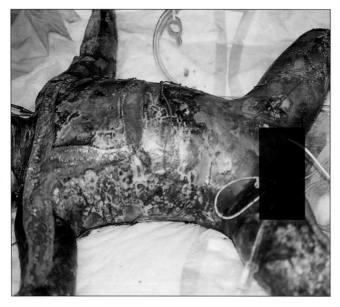

1.1.5.6 Ninety-nine percent full thickness burns after a gasoline explosion. Charred appearance is common to this agent.

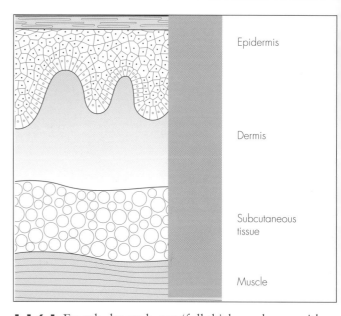

1.1.6.1 Fourth-degree burns (full thickness burns with involvement of deep structures). In this type of injury, extensive damage to deep structures, like muscle and bone, is present. Presentation is similar to that of third-degree burns, but extensive destruction of deep structures is also present.

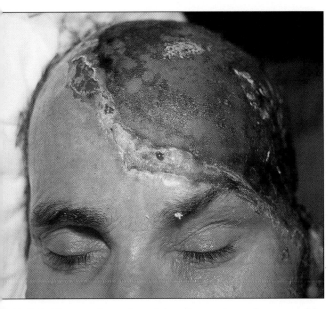

1.1.6.2 Contact burn involving the scalp and outer table of the skull. These burns carry a high mortality rate.

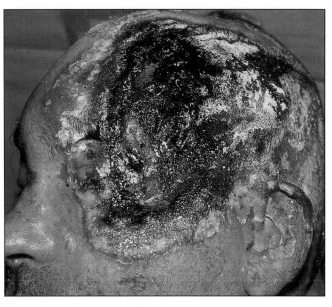

1.1.6.3 Fourth-degree burn involving muscle, eye ball, and outer table of the skull.

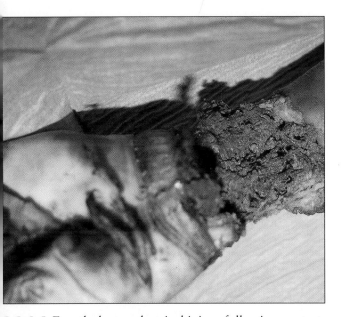

1.1.6.4 Fourth-degree electrical injury following contact with a high power wire. Note that all structures in the wrist have been destroyed.

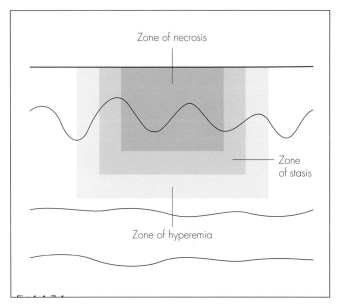

1.1.7.1 Zones of necrosis, stasis, and hyperemia corresponding to a partial thickness burn. If handled inappropriately, zone of stasis may convert to zone of necrosis; conversion to full thickness burns in these situations is possible. Increases in depth and horizontal extension of zone of necrosis, proportionally increases the zone of stasis and the chances of conversion to full thickness burn.

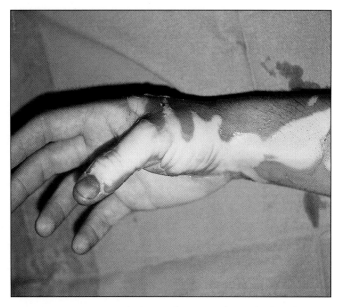

1.1.7.2 Deep second-degree burn to the right hand and forearm. Note the intense ischemic appearance of the injury.

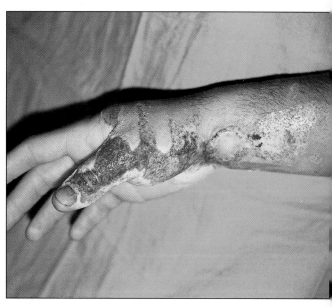

1.1.7.3 Same injury as in Figure 1.1.7.2, 24 hours later. Most of the ischemic and stasis zone has resolved with elevation and occlusive treatment with silver sulfadiazine. Wounds healed uneventfully in 15 days.

SYSTEMIC RESPONSES TO THERMAL INJURY

Burn Edema

Burn edema development during the first 24 hours	
Phase 1	High microvascular hydrostatic pressure Increase in transvascular fluid flux
Phase 2	Oncotic pressure gradient reduced Changes in microvascular permeability Important role of endothelial cells
Phase 3	Hyperdynamic cardiovascular response High filtration coefficient Increase in perfused area and pore numbers

1.2.1 The three phases of burn edema development. Burn edema is maximal between 24 and 48 hours after the injury, and resolves afterwards. Severe burns present with edema to burned and unburned tissues. It is important to remember that glottic edema may be present regardless of burn size and severity.

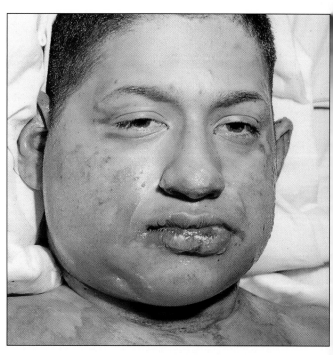

1.2.1.1 Intense edema to soft tissues of lower face 24 hours after a 21% total body surface area flame burn.

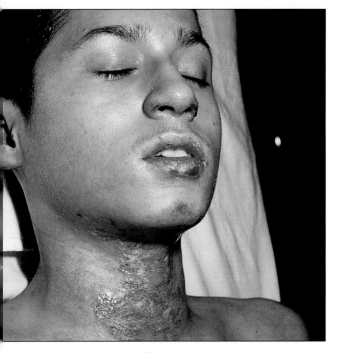

1.2.1.2 Same patient as shown in Figure 1.2.1.1 72 hours after the injury. All soft tissue edema has resolved. Elevation of all affected areas is essential to prevent edema and its complications.

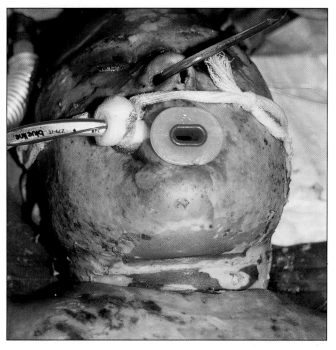

1.2.1.3 Severe edema to the face following 65% total body surface area burns in a gasoline tank explosion. Management of the airway with early prophylactic endotracheal intubation is paramount. Extubation 48–72 hours after the injury is normally feasible.

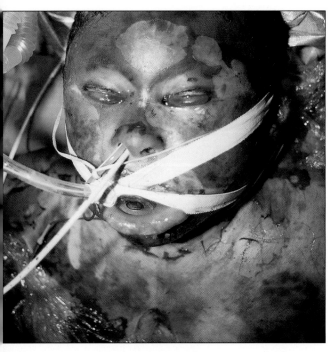

1.2.1.4 Patient with 85% full thickness burns. Edema to soft tissues is severe. Note that full thickness burns render the burned skin inelastic. In these circumstances pressure is transmitted to deep tissues, promoting compartment syndromes if left untreated. Note the intense edema to the conjunctivae and lower lip.

Systemic Effects

Systemic effects of the burn wound
• Systemic clotting derangements
• Decreased flexibility of red cells (heat damaged) and early destruction
• Suppression of cellular immunity
• Impairment of neutrophil function
• Peroxidation of hepatocytes
• Myocardial depression
• Hypermetabolism
• Multiple endocrine aberrations
• Renal tubule damage
• Decreased blood flow to the gut
• Pulmonary hypertension and edema
• Fat and skeletal muscle catabolism

1.2.2 Summarization of some of the major systemic effects of the burn wound.

SPECIFIC TYPES OF BURNS

Scald Burns

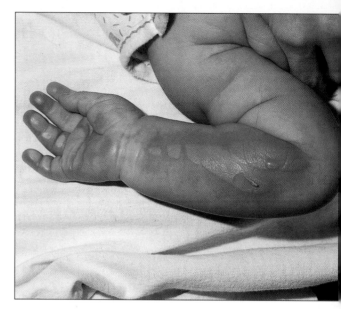

The systemic inflammatory response syndrome

- Body temperature >38°C or <36°C
- Heart rate > 90 beats/min
- Respiratory rate >20/min or $PaCO_2$ <32mmHg
- Leukocyte count >12000 µl, <4000 µl, or >10% immature (band) forms

1.2.3 Two or more of the conditions listed are necessary for the diagnosis of systemic inflammatory response syndrome (SIRS). Severe burns produce a SIRS that resembles sepsis. If the patient presents with any documented infection, SIRS becomes more profound, leading to septic shock if left untreated.

1.3.1.1 Superficial second-degree scald burn to the palm and forearm. Wounds healed in 7 days.

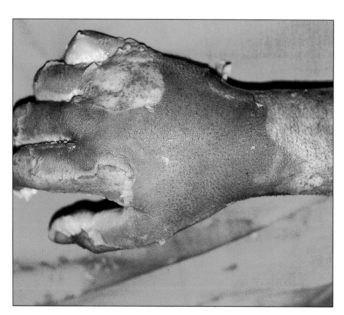

1.3.1.2 Deep second-degree scald injury to the right arm and dorsum of hand. Patient required excision and autografting.

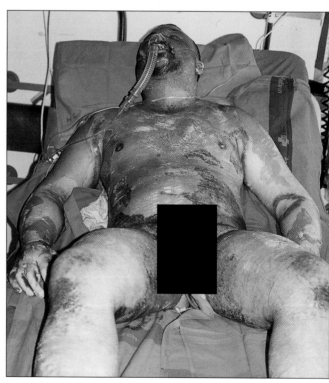

1.3.1.3 Ninety-five percent superficial and deep second-degree scald injury. The geographic appearance is typical of severe scalds, with a mixture of superficial and deep injuries in all affected areas.

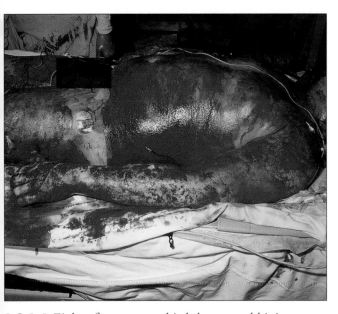

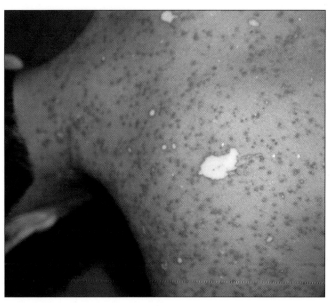

1.3.1.4 Eighty-five percent third-degree scald injury. Note the red appearance of all injuries, which can mislead a novice physician to consider these wounds second degree in nature. Hemoglobin is denatured and sequestered in all injured areas, giving the burns this otherwise typical appearance.

1.3.1.5 Splash scald with boiling oil. Note that injuries are deep second degree in nature.

Flame Burns

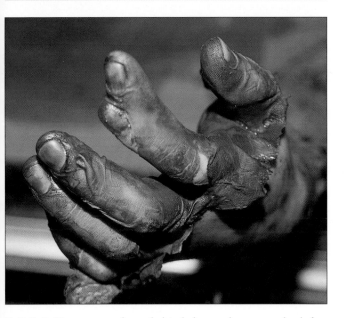

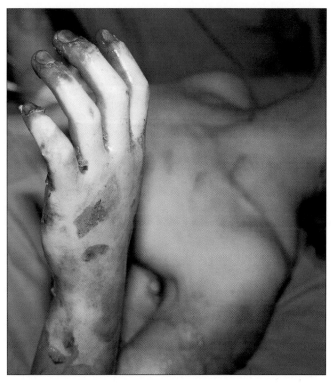

1.3.2.1 Deep second- and third-degree burns to the left arm caused by ignited gasoline. Heat produced with ignited gasoline is extremely intense, and extensive and deep injuries are therefore to be expected.

1.3.2.2 Appearance of the injuries in the same patient as shown in Figure 1.3.2.1 after removal of debris and dead skin.

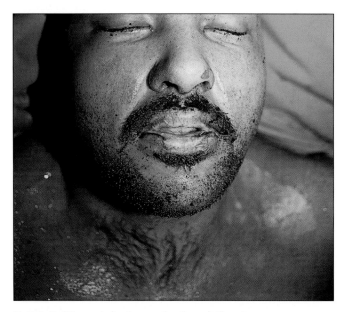

1.3.2.3 Flame injuries to the face following a gas explosion. Only exposed areas are likely to be burned in gas explosions, provided the clothes do not ignite. Trauma assessment should be focused also on associated injures that may occur after explosions.

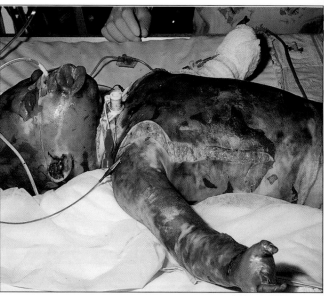

1.3.2.4 Eighty-five percent full thickness burns after a house fire. Flame injuries that occur in closed spaces are more prone to present with inhalation injury. Carboxyhemoglobin blood levels, cyanide blood levels, and bronchoscopy examination are very important in the diagnosis of inhalation injury.

Contact Burns

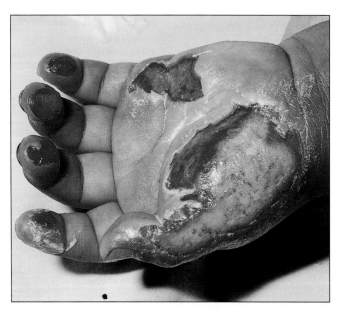

1.3.3.1 Deep second-degree contact burn with hot coals to the palm of a toddler. Contact burns that occur in young children and in the eldery tend to be full thickness because of the slow reactions in these populations. Other populations at risk are epileptic patients and substance abuse patients.

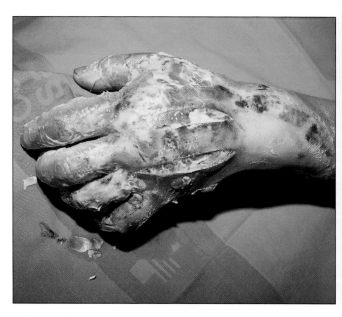

1.3.3.2 Contact burn with a space heater in an epileptic patient. Injury is full thickness in nature.

Chemical Burns

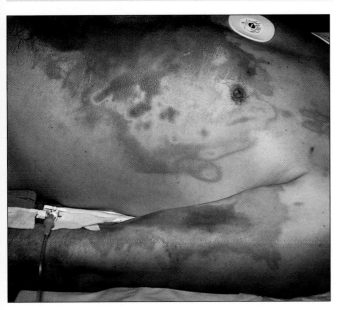

1.3.4.1 Full thickness burns after a work-related accident with nitric acid. Note the brownish appearance of these injuries, which is typical of chemical burns. Thorough irrigation with running water is the emergency local treatment. Immersion in a water bath is contraindicated because it can extend the injuries to normal skin by diluting the agent. Chemical antidotes should not be used because the reaction tends to be exothermic, adding a thermal component to the chemical component.

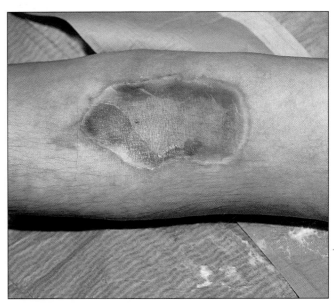

1.3.4.2 Alkali burn to the antecubital fossa. Burn are full thickness in nature.

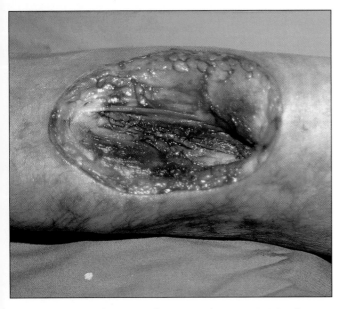

1.3.4.3 Same patient as shown in Figure 1.3.4.2 after removal of the superficial eschar. Denaturation of proteins progresses to deep tissues in chemical burns until the chemical agent is neutralized.

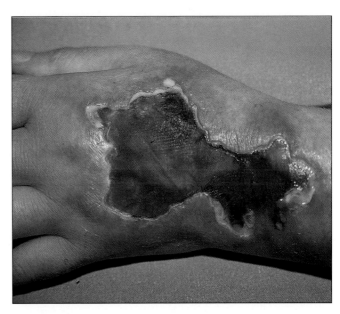

1.3.4.4 Extravasation of antineoplastic drug to the dorsum of the hand. These agents produce extensive local damage as chemical agents. The injury is full thickness in nature. All harmful drugs should be administered through central lines.

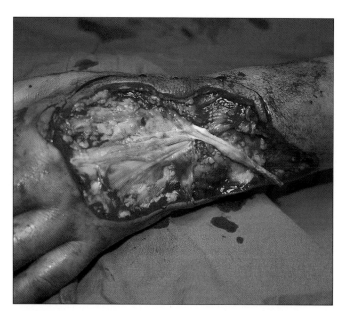

1.3.4.5 Same injury as shown in Figure 1.3.4.4 after removal of the superficial eschar. Note the extensive damage to the extensors and deep structures.

Molten Metals

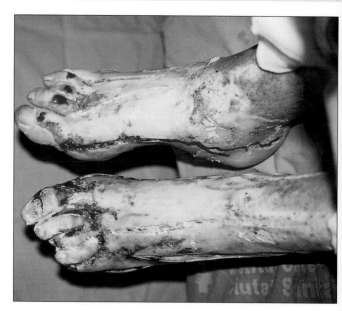

1.3.5.1 Molten zinc injuries to the feet after an industrial accident. Molten metals reach temperatures above 450°C. Injuries are full thickness in nature, and progress to fourth-degree injuries in the following days.

1.3.5.2 Final result after excision and debridement of all injured and devitalized tissues shown in Figure 1.3.5.1. Following all safety protocols at work is essential to prevent such injuries.

Electrical Burns

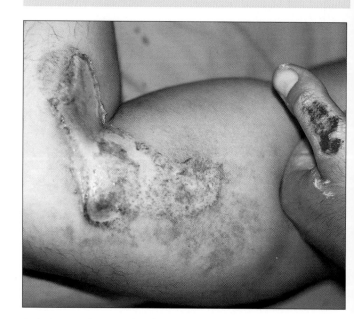

1.3.6.1 Voltaic arch after contact with a wire carrying 340V.

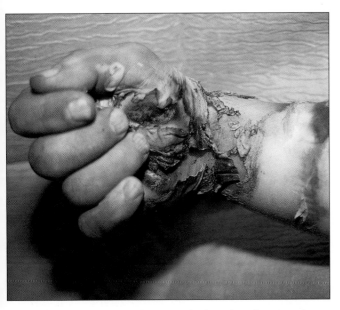

1.3.6.2 Fourth-degree burn to the hand and wrist after contact with a high power line. Note the claw deformity produced by the spastic contracture of flexor muscles. Compartment syndromes are likely to occur in such injuries, and exploration and fasciotomies are therefore mandatory.

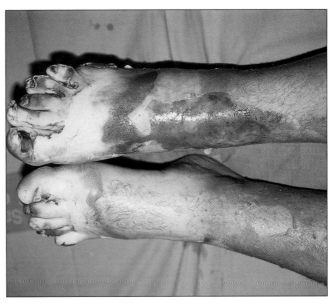

1.3.6.3 Exit wounds in the same patient as shown in Figure 1.3.6.2. Patient was standing grounded to the floor.

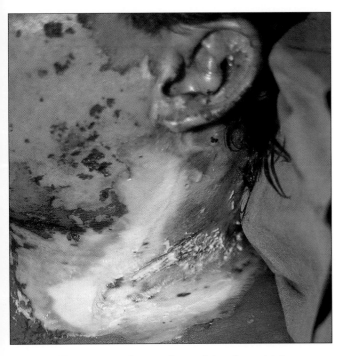

1.3.6.4 Entry wound to neck resulting from high power wire contact.

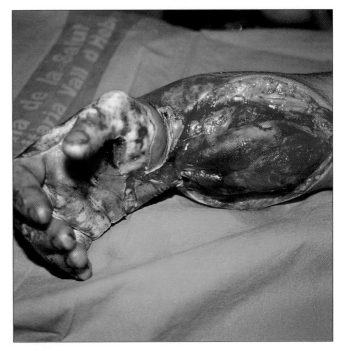

1.3.6.5 Fasciotomies are mandatory in compartment syndromes in electrical injuries. Note that muscles show some necrotic areas. Electrical injuries are often progressive for the next 2–3 days, so debridement in the first operation should be limited to grossly necrotic areas. Amputation may be needed in devastating injuries.

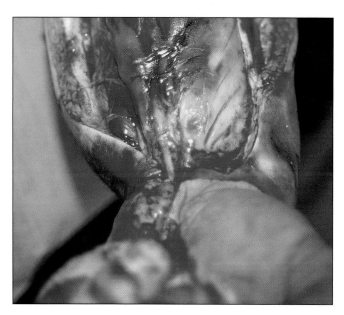

1.3.6.6 Close-up view of the injury shown in Figure 1.3.6.5, showing necrotic areas of the muscles and deep structures.

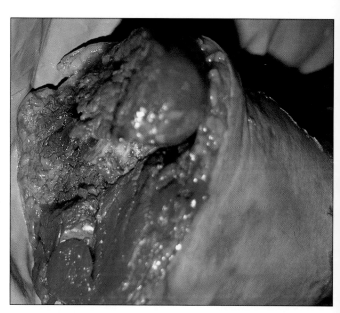

1.3.6.7 Close-up view of an amputated upper arm as definitive treatment for a severe massive electrical injury. Note that central compartment muscles are necrotic. Bone presents the highest resistance to the passage of electricity. Heat is produced and the maximum intensity of damage is in the deep structures. Injury follows a radial spread.

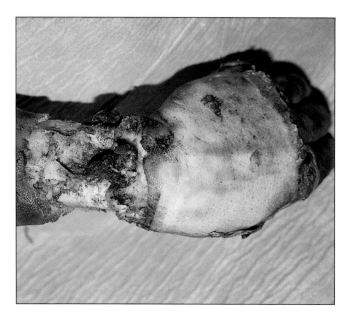

1.3.6.8 Complete destruction of the wrist after contact with a high power line. The hand is completely devascularized. A severe compartment syndrome can be noted in the forearm. Definitive treatment was amputation.

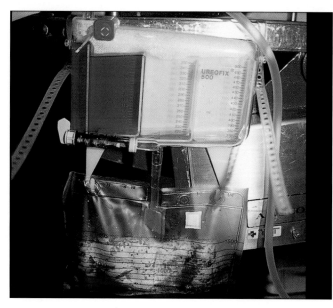

1.3.6.9 Myoglobinuria in a patient with high power electrical injuries. Urine output needs to be maintained above 100ml/h in adults until urine clears. Mannitol and alkalization of the urine is also helpful. Myoglobinuria, if left untreated, progresses to kidney damage and acute renal failure.

Firework Burns

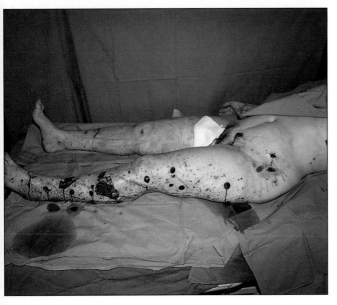

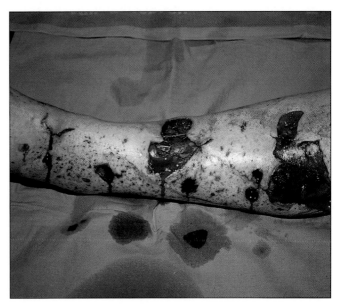

1.3.7.1 Powder grapeshot injuries after a firework explosion. Tracks need to be fully explored to rule out damage to deep structures. Injuries follow the pattern of low intensity gunshot. Secondary cavity formation is not likely to occur unless large fragments are involved.

1.3.7.2 Close-up of the same injury as shown in Figure 1.3.7.1. Long-term tattoo may occur.

SPECIFIC LOCATIONS

Upper Extremity Burns

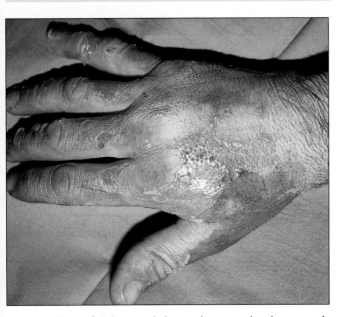

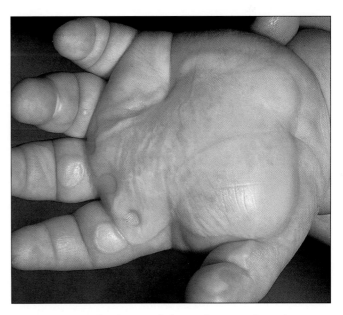

1.4.1.1 Superficial second-degree burn to the dorsum of the hand after a scald injury. Treatment with silver sulfadiazine or use of alternative coverings such as Biobrane is the correct treatment for these injuries. Elevation of the affected area is also very important.

1.4.1.2 Superficial second-degree burn to the palmar surface of the hand of a toddler. Child abuse should be considered in these injuries.

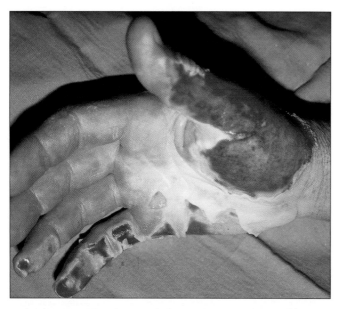

1.4.1.3 Superficial second-degree burn to the palmar surface of the hand of an adult. Appearance after blister removal.

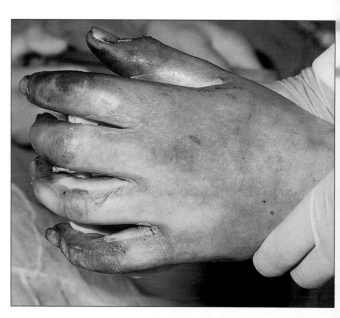

1.4.1.4 Superficial second-degree burns to the dorsum of the hand. Note that many times these injuries carry some components of deep second-degree burn. Care must be taken to prevent the progression of the zone of stasis to necrosis.

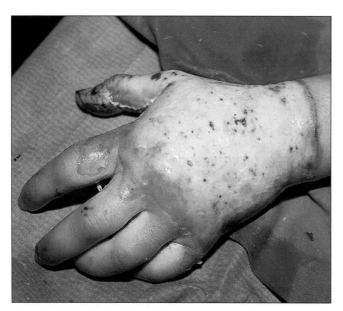

1.4.1.5 Deep second-degree burn to the dorsum of the hand. Flame injury with ignited alcohol. Note the edema to the dorsum of the hand and distally to the fingers. Proper wound care, elevation, and an assessment as to whether the wound will heal within 3 weeks are essential. Burns that do not present with the potential to heal within 3 weeks should be excised and autografted.

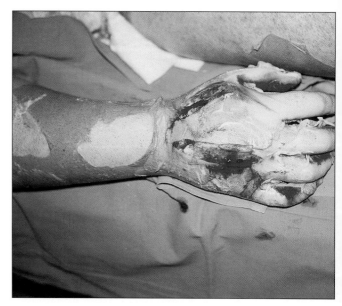

1.4.1.6 Full thickness burns to the hand and forearm. The inelastic eschar prevents the injured skin from expanding as edema develops. Escharotomies, therefore, are mandatory in all circumferential full thickness burns.

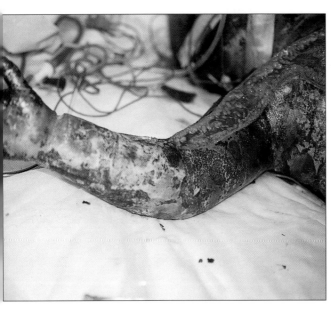

1.4.1.7 Third- and fourth-degree flame burns to the hand and upper extremity. Despite escharotomies, loss of fingers and limbs often results.

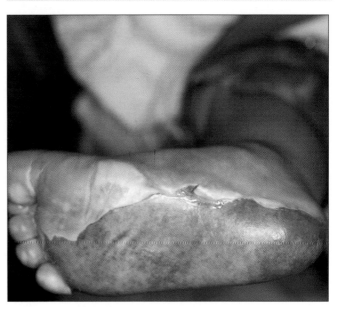

1.4.2.1 Superficial second-degree burn to the sole. Contact burns in small children often result in such injuries. Child abuse should be considered.

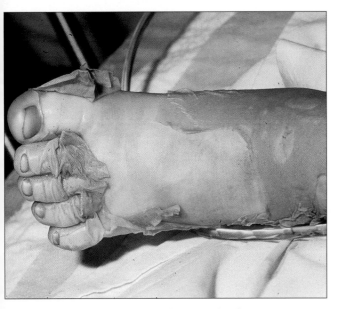

1.4.2.2 Deep second-degree burn to the foot. Excision and autografting are necessary.

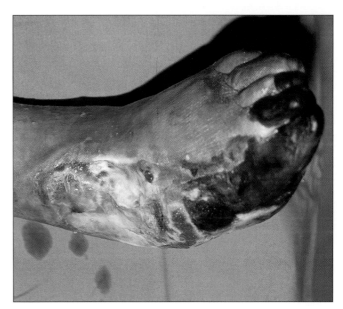

1.4.2.3 Full thickness contact burn to the foot. Contact burns can be locally devastating.

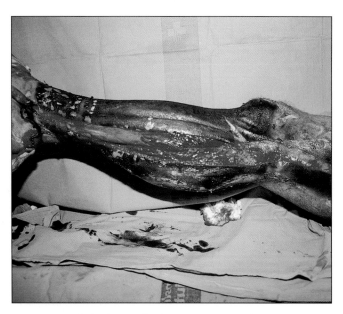

1.4.2.4 Full thickness flash injuries to the lower extremity. Note that escharotomies and fasciotomies were necessary to re-establish blood flow to the extremity.

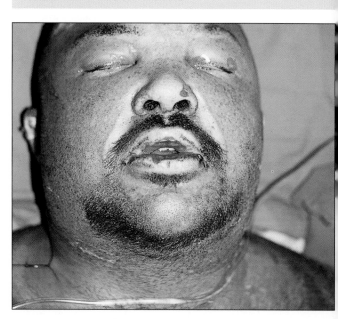

1.4.3.1 Superficial and deep second-degree burns to the face after a propane conflagration. Intense edema normally accompanies these injuries. Securing the airway is the first priority.

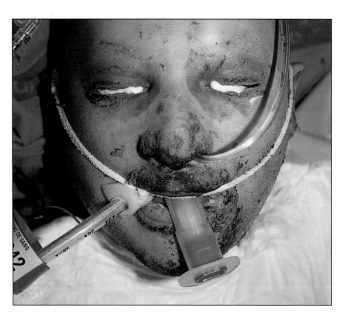

1.4.3.2 Full thickness burns to the face with ignited gasoline diluted with halogenates.

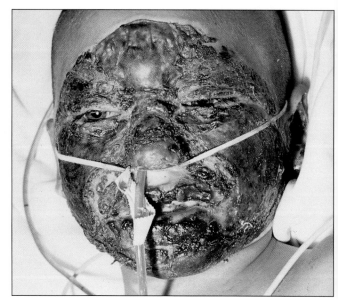

1.4.3.3 Full thickness flame injuries to the face. Appearance after 10 days using the exposure method of treatment.

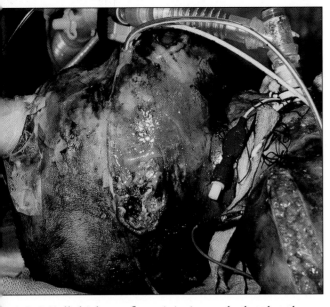

1.4.3.4 Full thickness flame injuries to the head and neck. The patient also suffered severe inhalation injury and thermal brain injury.

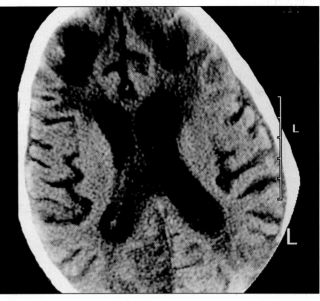

1.4.3.5 Computed axial tomography scan of the same patient as shown in Figure 1.4.3.4. Note the thermal lesions to the frontal and occipital lobes.

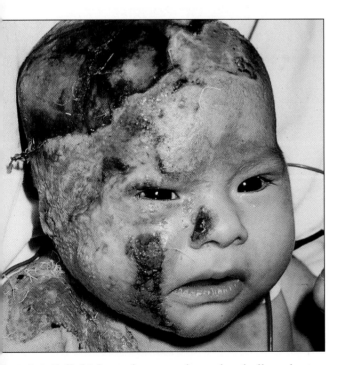

1.4.3.6 Full thickness burns to the scalp, skull, and brain in a 4-month-old infant. Diploë and internal and external tables are not developed at this age, so full thickness burns to bone result.

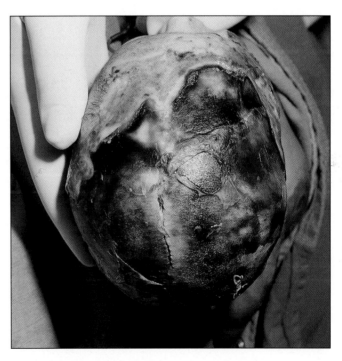

1.4.3.7 Axial view of the burns to the skull in the same patient as shown in Figure 1.4.3.6.

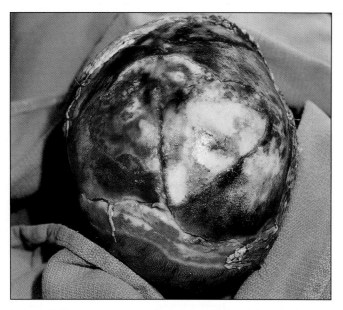

1.4.3.8 Same patient as shown in Figure 1.4.3.6 after partial craniectomy. Note that the meninges, brain, and sagittal sinus are burned and exposed.

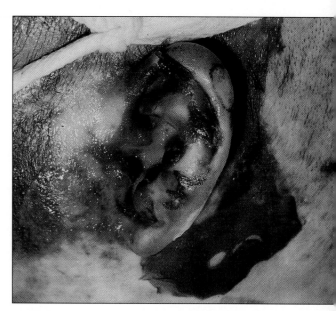

1.4.3.9 Full thickness burns to the ear. Pillows are to be avoided in all burns to the ears. Mafenide is very effective in the treatment of burns to the ears. Debridement should always be limited so that destruction and loss of parts of the ear is minimized.

SPECIAL TYPES OF INJURIES

Genital Burns

Hydrofluoric Acid Burns

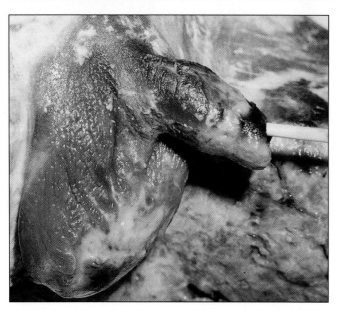

1.4.4.1 Burns to the penis and genitalia. Deep second-degree and third-degree burns are to be closely monitored. Such injuries may result in development of a compartmental syndrome. Penile loss may occur if a dorsal escharotomy to the penis is delayed. More localized injuries may result in paraphimosis.

General considerations and treatments in hydrofluoric acid burn injuries	
General considerations	• Systemic manifestation primarily takes the form of hypocalcemia • Patients with significant exposure need to be placed on cardiac monitors and have intravenous access obtained and serial determinations of electrolytes • Be prepared to administer large doses of intravenous calcium chloride • Rest of the initial care similar to that for any other chemical burn
Specific treatment	• Topical application of calcium gluconate-based gel • Subcutaneous injection of calcium gluconate • Intra-arterial infusions of calcium gluconate in digital and hand injuries

1.5.1 General considerations for hydrofluoric acid burns. Patients who have suffered significant exposure (either location or extension) should be admitted for specific treatment and monitoring.

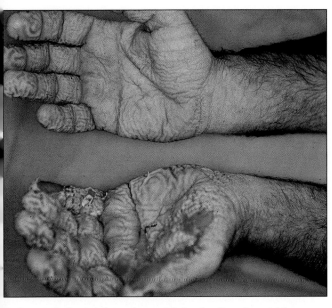

1.5.1.1 Industrial worker with hydrofluoric acid burns to both hands. Contact with skin causes excruciating pain.

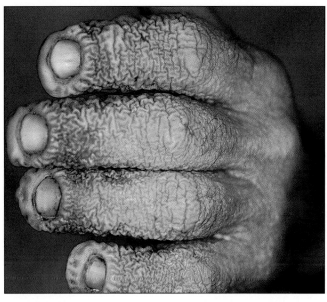

1.5.1.2 Maceration of the skin of the same patient shown in Figure 1.5.1.1, secondary to prolonged attempt at dilution of the acid with water. Dehydration and corrosion of tissue occurs, which is due to free H^+ ions.

Frostbite Injuries

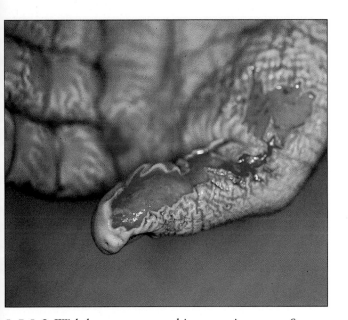

1.5.1.3 With long exposure, skin necrosis occurs. Seen here are areas of skin loss over the thenar eminence. Same patient as in Figure 1.5.1.1.

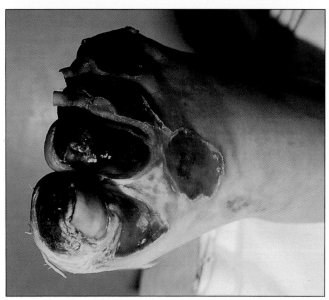

1.5.2 Cold-induced frostbite to the foot. Late appearance with necrosis of the toes. All frostbite cases, except for minor ones, should be admitted to a hospital. Rewarming is the initial treatment, followed by warm hydrotherapy, topical treatment with anti-inflammatory ointments, systemic oral ibuprofen, and debridement of blisters. Definitive treatment depends on the extent and depth of the injury.

Management of toxic epidermal necrolysis

- Debridement and application of biologic or synthetic dressings
- Avoid corticosteroid therapy
- Suspected drugs should be discontinued immediately
- Administration of pain medication and antipyretics is of high priority
- Consider empiric antibiotics if neutropenia exists
- Stress ulcer prophylaxis
- Administer oral nystatin
- Administer intravenous diphenhydramine
- Consider general treatment of any burn patient

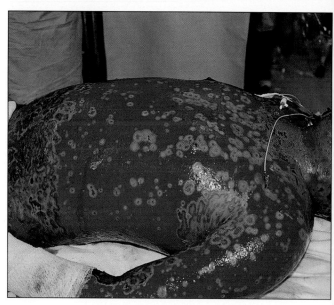

1.5.3 Toxic epidermal necrolysis is a life-threatening disease, and patients such as the one shown in Figure 1.5.3.1 are best managed in an intensive care burn unit where vigorous fluid resuscitation, nutritional support, wound care, physical therapy, and social services are routinely provided.

1.5.3.1 Toxic epidermal necrolysis in a young adult after phenytoin drug therapy. Note the islands of unaffected skin in the open wound. The patient suffered also from renal and mucosal involvement, with severe and life-threatening digestive bleeding that was controlled with Sengstaken-Blakemore balloon.

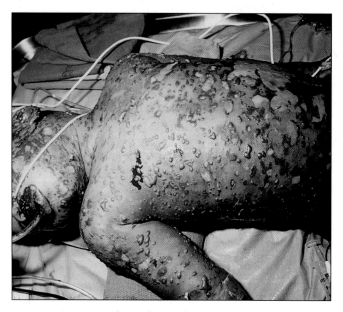

1.5.3.2 Toxic epidermal necrolysis in a 3-year-old male patient. Note the separation of the epidermis and the oral mucosa involvement.

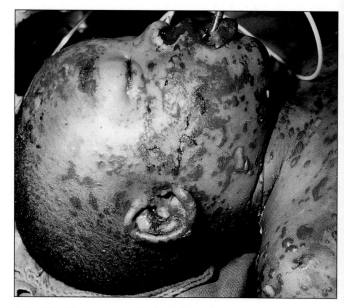

1.5.3.3 Close-up of the facial lesions shown in Figure 1.5.3.2. Vigorous debridement under anesthesia is necessary to peel off all the areas involved.

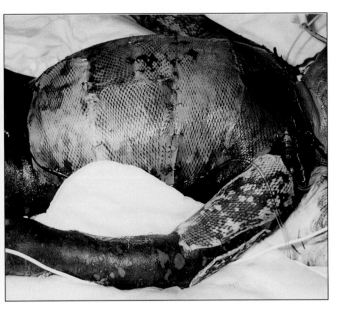

1.5.3.4 Treatment of the patient shown in Figure 1.5.3.2 included debridement, homografting, continuous intravenous drip of diphenhydramine, and general support.

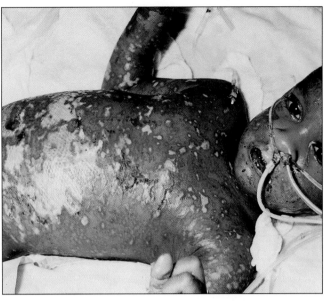

1.5.3.5 Same patient as shown in Figure 1.5.3.2 with all the wounds resolving. Homografting and intravenous diphenhydramine are very effective to stop the progression of the disease.

Abuse Injuries

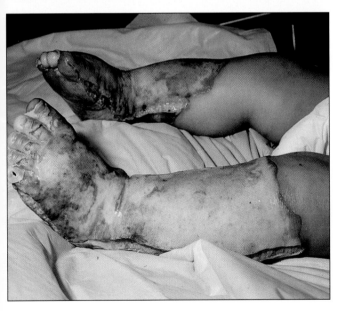

1.5.3.6 Immersion scald to the lower extremities in a 10-month-old male patient. Scalds with a clear line of delimitation are typical of child abuse injuries. Other signs of child abuse, such as wounds, fractures, old scars, bruises, supreme pain tolerance, and nutritional deficits, must be explored. In all suspicious injuries, further investigation and notification of child protective services should be carried out.

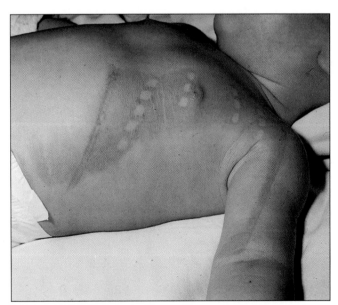

1.5.3.7 Contact iron burn. Note that the burn left an imprint of the iron on the child's skin, a typical characteristic of child abuse contact burns. Other populations at risk for abuse injuries include the elderly, the handicapped, and spouse abuse.

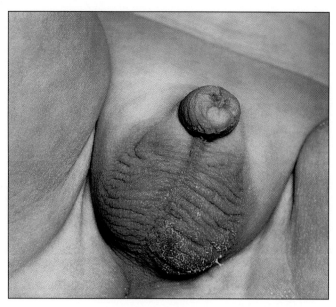

1.5.4 Cigarette burn to the genitalia of a 6-month-old baby.

CHAPTER 2
ORGANIZATION OF BURN CARE

David N. Herndon, MD and Juan P. Barret, MD

THE BURN TEAM

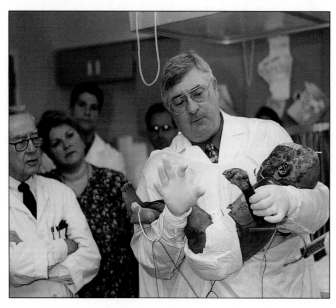

2.1 Different experts from diverse disciplines gather together with common goals and tasks, sharing overlapping values to achieve their objectives.

Main members of the burn team

- Burn surgeons (plastic surgeons and general surgeons)
- Nurses (intensive care unit acute and reconstructive wards, scrub nurses, anesthesia nurses)
- Case managers (acute and reconstructive)
- Anesthesiologists (experienced in burn anesthesia)
- Respiratory therapists
- Rehabilitation therapists
- Nutritionists
- Psychosocial experts
- Social workers
- Volunteers
- Microbiologists
- Research nurses
- Support services (secretarial services, environmental services, medical records, material management, informatics, technical services, etc.)

2.2 Main members of the burn team.

UTILIZATION AND COST-CONTAINMENT OF THE BURN CENTER

Patients suitable to be treated in a burn center

- Acute burn patients
- Rehabilitation and reconstructive burn patients
- Patients with toxic epidermal necrolysis and other life-threatening dermatoses
- Blunt and penetrating trauma patients
- Brain trauma patients
- Maxillofacial injury patients
- Upper and lower limb reconstruction patients
- Craniofacial surgery patients
- Free flap reconstruction patients
- Traumatic soft tissue avulsions
- Pressure sores
- Chronic wounds
- Diabetic and vascular ulcers

2.3 Burn patients (either in the acute or reconstructive phase), trauma patients, and plastic surgery patients are excellent candidates to be treated in burn centers. This improves their clinical care and the cost-efficiency of the center.

Priority of admissions to the burn center

Priority 1	• Severe burns • Electrical injuries • Burns with inhalation injury • Burns in infants • Burns in the elderly • Burns in patients with chronic or debilitating diseases • Toxic epidermal necrolysis
Priority 2	• Multiple blunt or penetrating trauma • Brain trauma • Maxillofacial injuries • Upper and lower limb reconstruction following trauma
Priority 3	• Free flap surgery • Craniofacial surgery • Other plastic surgery procedures

2.4 Priority of admissions to the burn center. Patients included in priority 1 have top priority for admission. If the center is full, priority 3 followed by priority 2 should be relocated, based on individual assessment. Priority 3 patients are admitted for elective surgery on the basis of availability of beds.

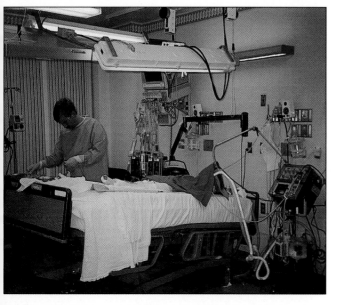

2.5 Burn intensive care unit room. Shriners Burns Hospital, Galveston. Spacious rooms are suitable for treatment of acute burn and trauma patients.

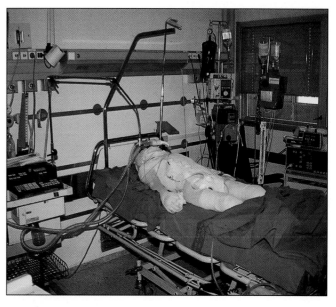

2.6 Burn intensive care unit room. Centre de Cremats de la Vall d'Hebron, Barcelona.

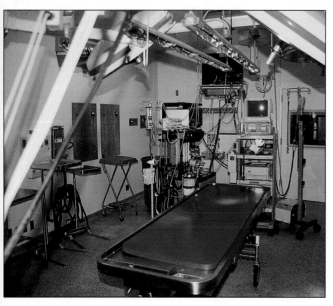

2.7 Burn operating room one. Shriners Burns Hospital, Galveston. Easy and direct access to the operating theater is very important in treating severe life-threatening burns.

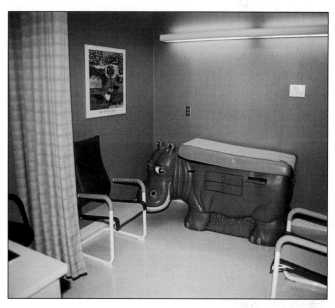

2.8 Integrated clinics in the burn center improve patient care and relationships among members of the burn team.

PATIENTS SUITABLE TO BE TREATED IN THE BURN CENTER

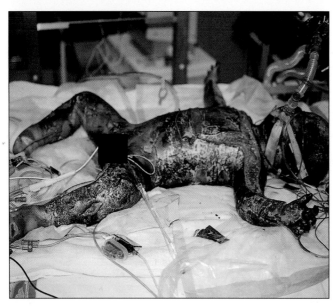

2.9 Priority 1 admission to a burn center. Ninety-nine percent, total body surface area, full thickness burns with severe inhalation injury.

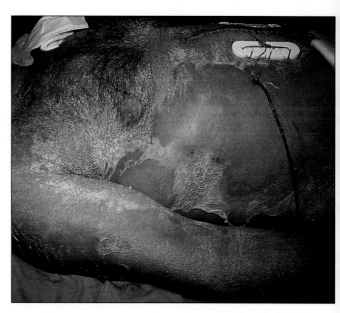

2.10 Erythrodermia in a patient with psoriasis. Life-threatening dermatoses are diseases that are best treated in the burn center.

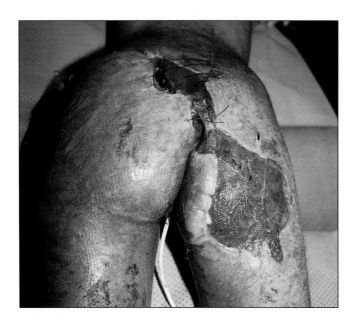

2.11 Multiple trauma after the patient was run over by a school bus. These patients can also be treated in the burn center by the burn team if the trauma team deems it appropriate.

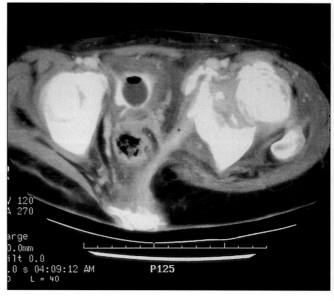

2.12 Computed tomography scan showing the internal injuries to the iliac bone, bladder, and rectum of the patient shown in Figure 2.11.

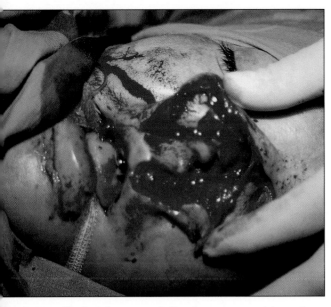

2.13 Maxillofacial trauma following a car accident. Seat belts were not fastened.

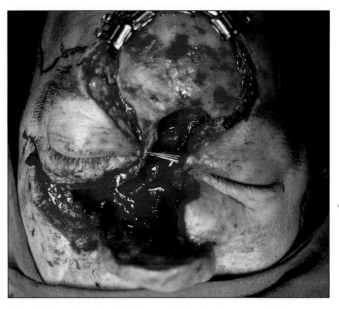

2.14 Complex facial injury following a motorbike collision. Patients with maxillofacial injuries can also be treated in the burn center. Skilled nurses, speech therapists, plastic surgeons, and dietitians can offer the best outcome for such patients.

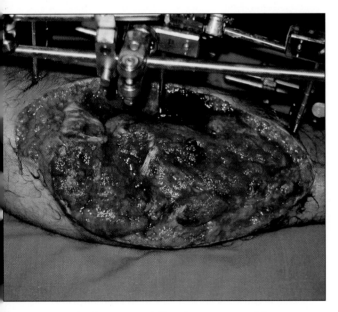

2.15 Lower limb trauma following a car accident. Wound care and closure can be accomplished by the burn team.

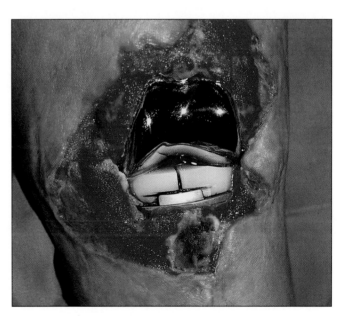

2.16 Lower limb reconstruction is also another pathology that can be treated, with good cost-efficiency.

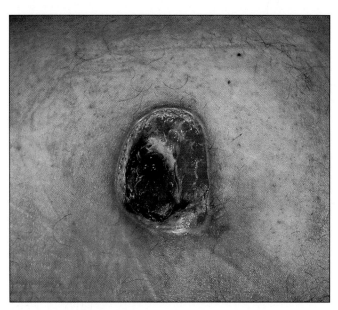

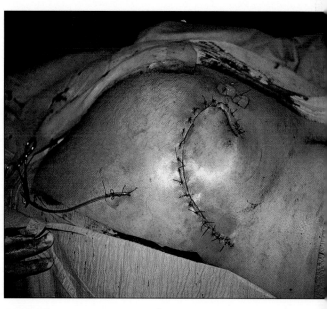

2.17 Gluteal pressure sore in a paraplegic patient. Patients affected by spinal cord injuries may be treated by burn center nurses, psychologists, plastic surgeons, and social workers.

2.18 The same patient as shown in Figure 2.17 after reconstruction with a rotational myocutaneous gluteal flap.

CHAPTER 3
INITIAL CARE AND RESUSCITATION

Juan P. Barret, MD and David N. Herndon, MD

PRIMARY AND SECONDARY ASSESSMENT

Primary assessment

- Administer 100% humidified oxygen
- Monitor respiratory status
- Endotracheal intubation if upper respiratory obstruction may develop
- Expose chest to assess ventilatory exchange (rule out circumferential burns)
- Assess ventilatory exchange after establishing a clear airway
- Assess blood pressure and pulse
- Accomplish cervical spine stabilization until the condition can be evaluated

3.1 Primary assessment guidelines. Immediate life-threatening conditions should be quickly identified and treated. The primary assessment is a rapid, systematic approach to identify life-threatening conditions.

Secondary assessment

- Thorough head-to-toe evaluation
- Careful determination of trauma other than obvious burn wounds
- Use cervical collars, backboards, and splits before moving the patient
- Examine past medical history, medications, allergies, and mechanism of injury
- If delay in transportation or estimation of transportation longer than 60 minutes, establish intravenous access and administer intravenous fluids
- Protect wounds from the environment with application of clean dressings
- Determine the needs for transportation. Contact receiving facility for further instructions

3.2 Secondary assessment guidelines. The secondary assessment is a more thorough head-to-toe evaluation of the patient. Initial management of a burned patient should be the same as for any other trauma patient.

Definitive assessment in the emergency department or burn center

- Primary assessment (see Fig. 3.1)
- Secondary assessment (see Fig. 3.2)
- Establish intravenous line and initiate resuscitation if not started on-site
- Establish history of the injury (mechanism, time, description of surrounding environment, enclosed space, presence of noxious chemicals, and possibility of smoke inhalation and any related trauma)
- Perform complete physical examination (with neurologic and corneal examinations)
- Examine extremities and record circumferential burns and pulses
- Perform escharotomies if needed
- Evaluate wounds
- Estimate burn size and depth
- Laboratory tests

3.3 A final assessment of the patient is performed at the receiving facility. It includes the primary and secondary assessment, and a final diagnosis and establishment of a plan of care.

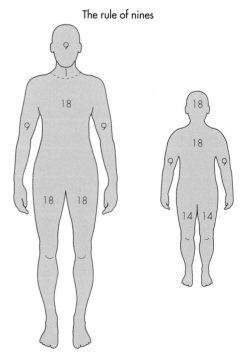

The rule of nines

3.4 An easy and quick way to estimate the burn size is to use the 'rule of nines'. A better and more accurate estimation must be accomplished as soon as possible by using more accurate tables such as the Lund and Browder chart (see Figure 11.1)

Escharotomies of chest and upper extremities

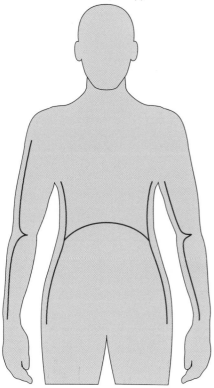

3.5 Suggested placement of escharotomies to the chest and upper extremities. Note that darts should be included so that linear hypertrophic scars do not result.

Escharotomies of lower extremities

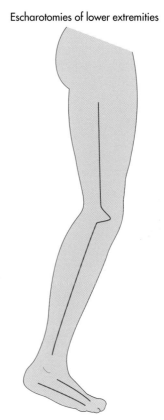

3.6 Lower extremity escharotomies. Fasciotomies need to be considered if compartment syndromes are present.

Escharotomies of hands

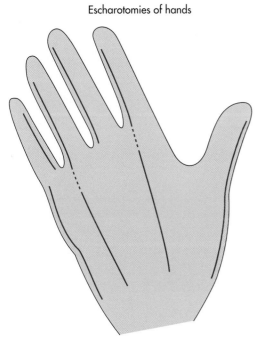

3.7 Hand escharotomies. Thenar, hypothenar, and interosseous compartments should be explored if high pressures are noted. Carpal and Guyon tunnel releases may be considered in severe injuries with neural compromise.

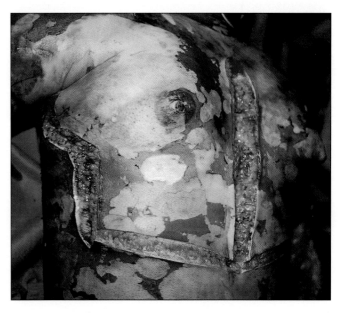

3.8 Chest escharotomies in full thickness burns.

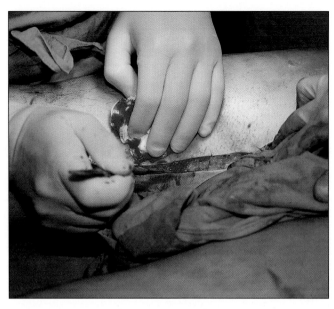

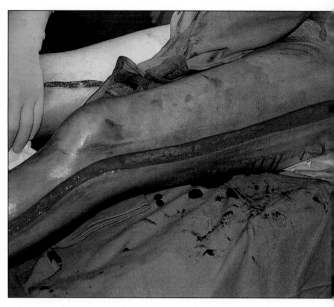

3.9 Lower limb escharotomy. The knife or Bovie may be used. Excessive bleeding may occur with the use of knife blades, whereas use of the Bovie can result in more pain in patients without deep sedation.

3.10 The same patient as shown in Figure 3.9, with escharotomies completed. Note that only the eschar has been transected. Subcutaneous tissue should not be included in the escharotomy. If excessive pressure is still noted, a blunt fasciotomy may be required.

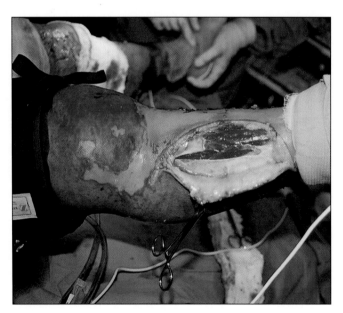

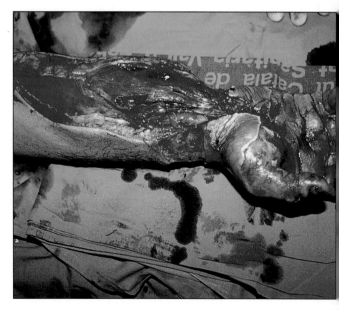

3.11 Fasciotomies in severe full thickness burns.

3.12 Fasciotomies in upper limb, high voltage electrical injuries.

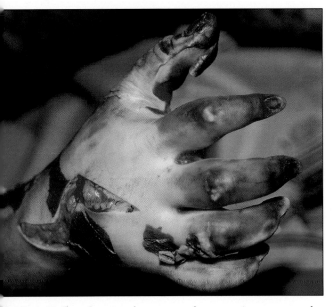

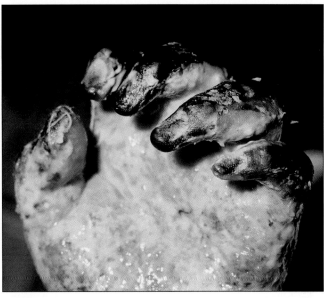

3.13 A Delayed or inadequate escharotomies may result n necrosis of digits, muscle compartments, or limbs. Note the necrosis of the fingers following inadequate escharotomies.

3.13 B Necrosis of the fingers after delayed resuscitation and inadequate escharotomies.

RESUSCITATION

Guidelines for correct resuscitation

- Do not delay resuscitation
- Estimate burn size and calculate fluid requirements
- Fluid formulas are only a guideline; monitor urine output and tailor intravenous fluids to the response of the patient
- Monitor peripheral pulses, blood pressure, respiration rate, heart rate, urine output, oxygen saturation, and temperature
- Monitor central venous pressure and/or cardiac output and hemodynamic parameters in severe burns or patients at risk for complications
- Achieve a urine output of 0.5ml/kg per h in adults and 1ml/kg per h in children – **no more, no less!**
- Elevate the head, limbs, and genitalia; elevate all that can be elevated
- Maintain the core temperature of the patient over 37°C
- Start enteral feeding on admission
- The aim is to maintain an awake, alert, conscious and cooperative patient
- Do not obtain a replica of the Michelin Man

3.14 Guidelines for correct resuscitation. The aim is to have a lucid and alert patient with good urine output. Over- and under-resuscitation may result in serious complications.

Recommended fluid formulas

Pediatric patients

Lactated Ringer's – add albumin 25% solution to maintain serum albumin >2.0g/dl

Add D5W in children under 2 years old

Add 1000ml/m^2 body surface area if in Clinitron bed

First 24h:
5000ml/m^2 body surface area burned
2000ml/m^2 body surface area
(50% in the first 8h and the subsequent 50% in the remaining 16h)

Subsequent 24h:
3750ml/m^2 body surface area burned
1500ml/m^2 body surface area

Adult patients

Lactated Ringer's

Add 1000ml/m^2 body surface area if in Clinitron bed

Modified Parkland formula:

3ml/kg for each per cent of total body surface area burned

(50% in the first 8h and the subsequent 50% in the remaining 16h)

3.15 Resuscitation formulas for pediatric and adult burn patients. Remember that these are only guidelines. Resuscitation must be tailored to each patient, and increased or decreased based on urine output and the clinical picture.

Monitoring of the burn patient

- Continuous electrocardiographic monitoring
- Continuous respiratory rate monitoring
- Pulse-oximetry
- Central venous pressure
- Arterial line
- Foley catheter and urine output
- Temperature probes
- Capnometry (ventilated patients)
- Swan-Ganz catheter (unstable severe burn patients)
- Doppler monitor for compartmental syndromes

3.16 Essential monitoring of the burn patient.

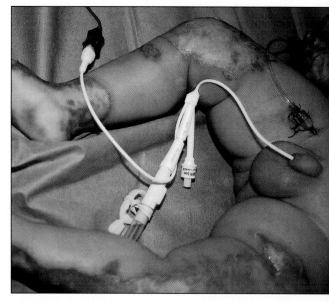

3.17 Core temperature monitoring via Foley catheters. Maintaining core temperatures over 37°C is essential for good resuscitation.

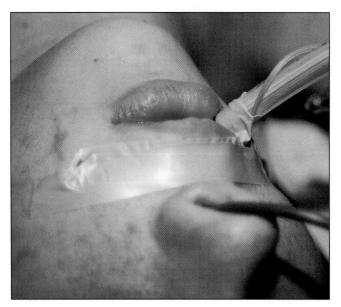

3.18 Rectal, nasal, or esophageal temperature probes are also of value for temperature monitoring. Note the nasal probe in this patient.

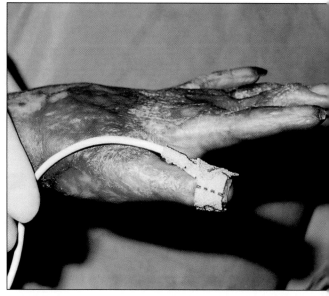

3.19 Pulse-oximeters are also very important during resuscitation and monitoring of burn patients. A wide range of different types of devices is currently available. Maintaining a high oxygen tension is essential to maintain tissue viability.

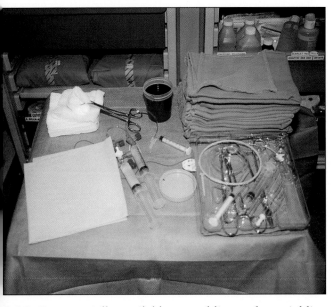

3.20 Commercially available central line and arterial line kits are very helpful for quick and safe line placement. Different widths and lengths are available to fit patient requirements.

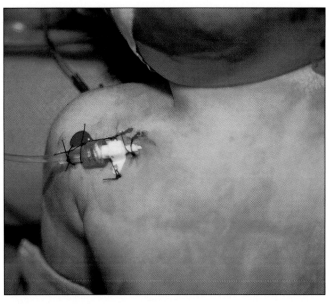

3.21 Subclavian line in place. Shoulder roles are very helpful in pediatric patients.

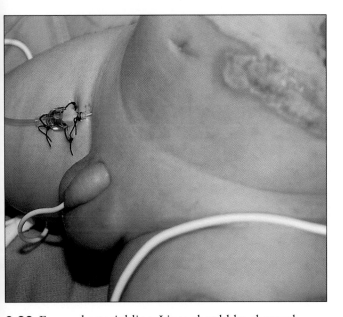

3.22 Femoral arterial line. Lines should be changed using a wire every 3 days. A new line should be placed with a new stick after a week in order to prevent catheter sepsis.

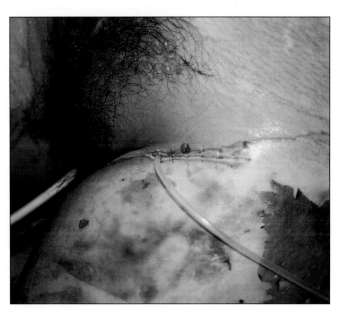

3.23 Cut-downs and burned tissue should be avoided for line placement. Risk of thrombosis and thrombophlebitis is high in these circumstances. If all areas are burned, excision of the area and placement of the catheter afterwards is advisable. Resuscitation must be started, however, via a large-bore catheter through burned tissue while the new catheter is being placed.

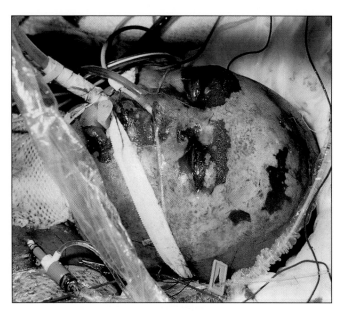

3.24 Swan–Ganz catheter in a patient with an 80% total body surface area full thickness burn and inhalation injury.

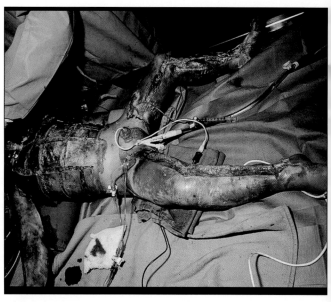

3.25 Monitoring of a burn patient. Note the temperature probe Foley, arterial line, central line, and pulse-oximeter. Enteral nutrition has been started and escharotomies performed.

TRANSPORTATION

Criteria for transfer to a burn center

- Second- and third-degree burns over 10% total body surface area in children <10 years or adults >50 years of age
- Second- and third-degree burns over 20% total body surface area at any age
- Third-degree burns over 10% total body surface area in any age group
- Second- and third-degree burns that involve the face, hands, genitalia, perineum, and major joints functionally or cosmetically
- Chemical burns
- Electrical burns, including lightning injuries
- Second- and third-degree burns with concomitant trauma in which the burn injury poses the greatest risk to the patient
- Burns with inhalation injury
- Patients with pre-existing medical disorders that could adversely effect patient care and outcome
- Hospitals without qualified personnel or equipment for the care of critically burned children

3.26 Criteria for transfer of a burn patient to a burn center.

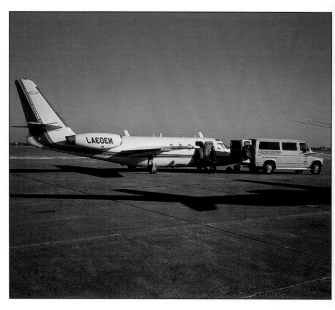

3.27 Fixed wing aircraft are the preferred transportation mode for critical burn patients at the Shriners Burns Hospital, Galveston.

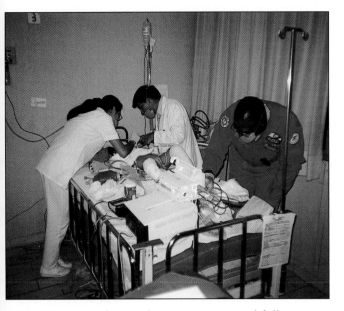

3.28 Primary and secondary assessment and full monitoring of the patient are mandatory before transportation.

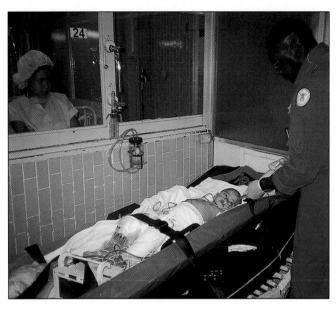

3.29 Patient ready for transportation.

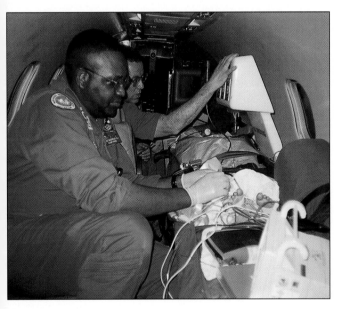

3.30 Portable monitors and ventilators are essential for correct monitoring. In many cases a team, including a physician, nurse, and respiratory therapist, is necessary.

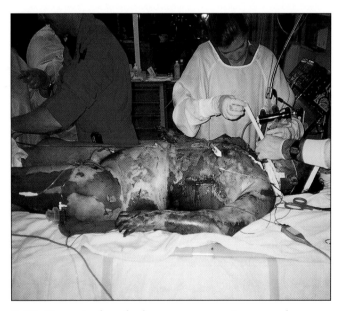

3.31 On arrival to the burn center, a primary and secondary assessment, final diagnosis, bronchoscopy, and formal resuscitation must be done.

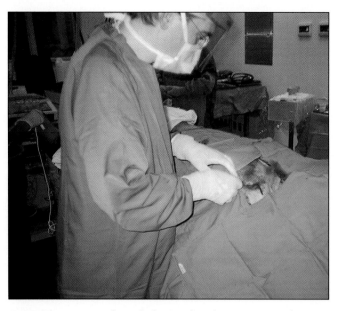

3.32 Placement of a subclavian line by a registered nurse anesthetist after arrival at the burn center.

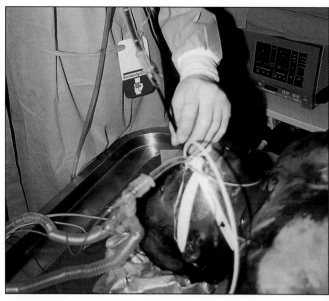

3.33 Direct bronchoscopy is essential for the diagnosis of inhalation injury. Note that an endotracheal tube has been placed on the bronchoscope in case a nasal intubation is necessary.

NUTRITIONAL SUPPORT

Initial nutritional assessment

- Determine the caloric and protein needs of a patient immediately upon admission
- Assessment by physician and dietitian
- Assess:
  Personal background
  Chronic conditions
  Hypermetabolic conditions
  Physical conditions that may interfere with food intake
  Predisposing factors
  Recent weight loss or gain
  Food preference and allergies
  Weight and height for age and sex
  Total lymphocyte count
  White blood cells
  Hemoglobin and hematocrit
  Mean corpuscular volume
- Perform indirect colorimetry if available
- Calculate daily calorie and protein needs

3.34 Patients should be assessed for nutritional status on admission, and nutritional needs should be reassessed on a daily basis. Inadequate intake necessitates an alteration of the regimen. It is also important to determine whether the regimen is well tolerated.

Factors that affect metabolic rate

- Keep environmental temperature at 33°C with low humidity
- Frightening and painful procedures should be kept to a minimum
- Utilize occlusive dressings to decrease evaporative water loss
- Perform dressing changes quickly and efficiently to avoid intermittent hypothermia resulting in 'cold stress'

3.35 Different factors can affect the metabolic rate. If these are not controlled, severe muscle and fat wasting may result.

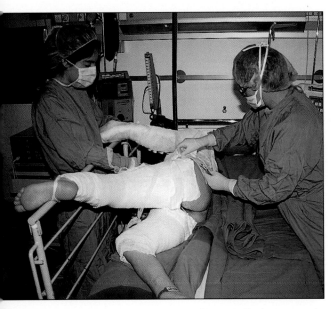

Nutritional formulas for pediatric burn patients	
0–12 months	2100kcal/m^2 surface area 1000kcal/m^2 surface area burn
1–11 years	1800kcal/m^2 surface area 1300kcal/m^2 surface area burn
≥12 years	1500kcal/m^2 surface area 1500kcal/m^2 surface area burn

3.37 Nutritional formulas for pediatric burn patients used at Shriners Burns Hospital, Galveston.

3.36 Experienced nurses with excellent skills for wound care are necessary in order to diminish time of dressing changes.

Nutritional formulas for adult burn patients	
16–59 years	25kcal/kg + 40kcal for each percent of burn
≥60 years	20kcal/kg + 65kcal for each percent of burn

3.38 Nutritional formulas for adult burned patients used at the University of Texas Medical Branch, Galveston.

Protein needs	
Birth to 0.5 years	4.4g/kg
0.5–2.0 years	4.0g/kg
2.0 years to adult	120:1 (kcal:N)

3.39 Protein needs in burn patients at different ages.

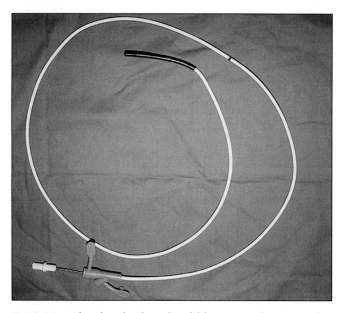

3.40 Nasoduodenal tubes should be inserted on arrival at the burn center and enteral nutrition started after the patient has been stabilized. Nutrition absorbed by the patient needs to be subtracted from the resuscitation needs.

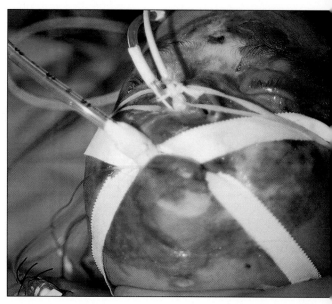

3.41 Enteral tubes must be securely fixed. Note that the patient has a nasogastric tube and a nasoduodenal tube in place. Of nutritional needs 10% are given through the nasogastric tube. At hourly intervals, gastric residues are checked via the nasogastric tube. If residue is higher than a 2 h enteral nutrition load, nutrition needs to be stopped and the cause investigated. Tube misplacement and sepsis are the most common causes of nutrition intolerance.

MANAGEMENT OF PAIN, ANXIETY, ITCH, AND STRESS DISORDERS

Guidelines for pain management in burn patients
• If the patient says he/she has pain, then he/she has pain
• Analgesics are most effective when given on a regular basis
• Intramuscular injections are not usually appropriate because the patient fears the injection as much as the pain
• Bowel management begins with narcotic pain management
• Pain medications should be individualized in the first 48h after burn, according to respiratory difficulty, septic shock, and malnutrition

3.42 Guidelines for pain management in burn patients.

The faces pain-rating scale

0   1   2   3   4   5

3.43 The faces pain-rating scale. The patient points to one of the faces that best expresses his/her pain status. (Adapted from the Varni Thompson pediatric pain questionnaire)

The observer pain scale	
Score 1	Patient laughing, euphoria
Score 2	Patient happy, smiling, playing
Score 3	Neutral (asleep or calm)
Score 4	Mild–moderate pain: expresses, vocalizes pain (whincing, etc.)
Score 5	Moderate–severe pain: crying, screaming, sobbing

3.44 The observer scale is used in children who are preverbal or who communicate nonverbally. In those patients with decreased levels of consciousness, pain cannot be assessed with these scales. Level of consciousness, however, should be noted on the vital sign flow sheet. Adapted with permission from Broadman *et al.*

Background pain management protocol	
Begin with acetaminophen (paracetamol)	15mg/kg per dose orally q4h
If pain is not controlled add morphine	0.03mg/kg per dose intravenously q4h 0.1–0.3mg/kg per dose orally q4h
Do not give morphine if patient asleep; do not give morphine for anxiety; do not give morphine if patient in shock or septic; do not give morphine if patient is not monitored	
Taper narcotics over 3 days	

Other drugs
  Levodromoran
 	
  Ibuprofen
	
	2mg orally q6–24h PRN (patients >16 years old)
	10mg/kg per dose orally q4h

3.45 Background pain management.

Procedural pain management
• Schedule pain medication 30min to 1h before procedure
• An anxiolytic with amnestic properties should be given in conjunction with the pain medication
• Doses of pain medications
Acetaminophen (paracetamol; if opiates not needed): 15mg/kg per dose
Morphine PO 0.3–0.6mg/kg per dose
IV 0.05–0.1mg/kg per dose
Fentanyl oralet 10µg/kg per dose rounded to nearest 100
• Doses of anxiolytic medication
Lorazepam IV or PO 0.05/kg per dose
Midazolam IV 0.05mg/kg per dose
PO 0.5mg/kg per dose up to a maximum of 20mg

Major dressing change or procedure

• **Children:** Ketamine IV 1–2mg/kg per dose
              IM 3–7mg/kg per dose
              PO 6–10mg/kg per dose
• **Adults:** Ketamine IV 1–2mg/kg per dose, titrate to effect
              IM 3–8mg/kg per dose
    Add benzodiazepines in conjunction with ketamine in adults
• **Propofol (adults and children):** 1.5–2mg/kg per dose IV (produces unconsciousness within 30s; titrate to maintain spontaneous ventilation)
• **Nitrous oxide**
• **Patients receiving conscious sedation need full monitoring**

3.46 Procedural pain management. IM, intramuscular; IV, intravenous; PO, orally.

Anxiety management in burn patients	
Before using anxiolytics, address pain management and acute stress disorder problems	
Lorazepam	0.03mg/kg per dose, I.V. or orally q4h
Diazepam	0.1mg/kg per dose, intravenously or orally q8–12h
Taper lorazepam in patients receiving the drug for more than 15 days; diazepam useful in rehabilitation (relaxes skeletal muscle)	

3.47 Anxiety management in burn patients.

Management of itch in burn patients	
Use moisturizing body shampoo and lotions to alleviate dry scaly skin	
Diphenhydramine	1.25mg/kg per dose orally q6h
Hydroxyzine	0.5mg/kg per dose orally q6h
Cyproheptadine	0.1mg/kg per dose orally q6h
Loratidine (children over 6 years of age)	10mg "

3.48 Management of itch due to inflammatory response in burn scar area.

Management of acute stress disorder and post-traumatic stress disorder	
Imipramine	1mg/kg per dose (advance dose based on levels or PR interval; draw IV levels starting 1 week after imipramine is begun)

Fluoxetine
  for patients ≤40kg
  for patients >40kg and ≤60kg
  for patients >60kg
	5mg
	10mg
	20mg

3.49 Management of acute stress disorder and post-traumatic stress disorder.

CHAPTER 4
INHALATION INJURY AND RESPIRATORY CARE

Lynn A. 'Pete' Peterson, CRNA, MSN; Ronald P. Mlcak, RRT; Juan P. Barret, MD; Ray J. Nichols Jr, MD

TOXIC SMOKE COMPOUNDS

Toxic smoke compounds

- Carbon monoxide and corbon dioxide
- Aldehydes and acrolein (cellulose combustion)
- Hydrogen cyanide, ammonia, hydrogen sulfide (wool and silk combustion)
- Sulfur dioxide, hydrogen sulfide (rubber combustion)
- Hydrogen chloride, phosgene (polyvinyl chloride combustion)
- Hydrogen cyanide, isocyanates, ammonia, acrylonitriles (polyurethane combustion)
- Hydrogen chloride (polyester combustion)
- Acrolein (polypropylene combustion)
- Hydrogen cyanide (polyacrylonitrile combustion)
- Hydrogen cyanide, ammonia (polyamide combustion)
- Hydrogen cyanide, ammonia, formaldehyde (melamine resins combustion)
- Acrolein (acrylics combustion)

4.1 Approximately 80% of fire-related deaths result not from burn injury but from inhalation of the toxic products of combustion. Most of these compounds are produced by combustion of clothing, fabrics, appliances, furniture, and household and kitchen goods.

Symptoms and signs of carboxyhemoglobin intoxication

Carboxhemoglobin level (%)	Symptoms
0–10	None
11–20	Tightness over forehead, slight headache, dilatation of cutaneous blood vessels
21–30	Headache and throbbing in the temples
31–40	Severe headache, weakness, dizziness, dimness of vision, nausea, vomiting, collapse
41–50	As above; greater possibility of collapse, syncope and increased pulse and respiratory rate
51–60	Syncope, increased pulse and respiratory rate, coma, intermittent convulsions, Cheyne–Stokes respirations
61–70	Coma, intermittent convulsions, depressed cardiac and respiratory function, possible death
71–80	Weak pulse, slow respirations, death within hours
81–90	Death in less than 1h
91–100	Death within minutes

4.2 Carbon monoxide toxicity remains one of the most frequent immediate causes of death following smoke-induced inhalation injury; it must be suspected in every fire victim and treated promptly. Inhalation of a 0.1% carbon monoxide mixture may result in generation of a carboxyhemoglobin level as high as 50%.

PATHOPHYSIOLOGY OF INHALATION INJURY

Injury to the oropharynx

- Heat denaturation of protein
- Complement activation
- Histamine release
- Conversion of xanthine oxidase
- Release of superoxide ion
- Permeability changes and neutrophil adherence

4.3 Sequence of changes that occur in the oropharynx as a result of thermal injury. The damage seen in this area after inhalation injury is the same as that seen with thermal injury in other areas of the body. The massive edema that results in the soft tissue of the oropharynx after burns, involves most of the variables in the Starling equation.

Airway pathophysiology in inhalation injury

- Irritants in smoke stimulate sensory nerves of the airway
- Release of neuropeptides (substance P and calcitonin gene-related peptides)
- Bronchial vasodilatation and increase in bronchovascular permeability
- Airway edema and/or cast formation with subsequent airway narrowing or obstruction

4.4 Sequence of events that lead to the airway pathophysiology associated with smoke inhalation. These changes in microvascular fluid flux occur with the elevation of polymorphonuclear cells, such as proteases and oxygen free radicals.

Pulmonary parenchymal injury
• Damage to the airway
• Release of mediators into bronchial venous drainage
• Upregulation of adherence molecules on pulmonary microvascular endothelial cells
• Adherence of neutrophils to endothelium
• Release of oxygen free radicals and proteases by neutrophils
• Increased pulmonary microvascular permeability
• Pulmonary edema and alveolar collapse

4.5 Sequence of events that lead to pathophysiology in the pulmonary microvascular areas. The delayed onset of the changes in transvascular fluid flux in the pulmonary bed suggests the release of mediators from other areas.

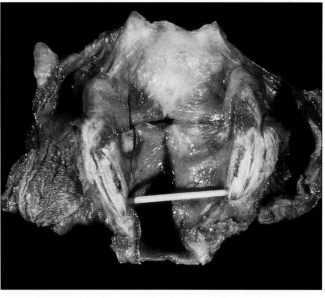

4.6 Inhalation injury to the true and false cords. Note the edema and erosion to the mucosa.

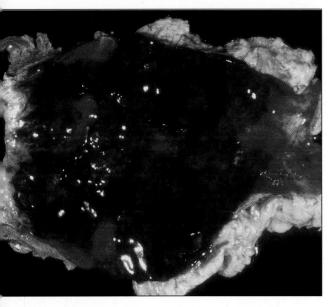

4.7 Severe inhalation injury to the larynx. Note the necrohemorrhagic changes to all of the structures involved in the process.

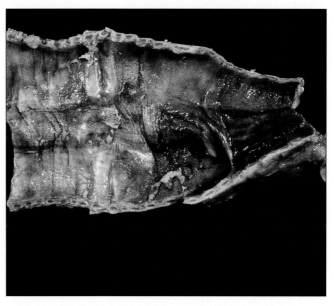

4.8 Injury to the trachea and main bronchi following severe inhalation injury. The inflammatory process usually extends beyond the upper airway with secondary airway damage.

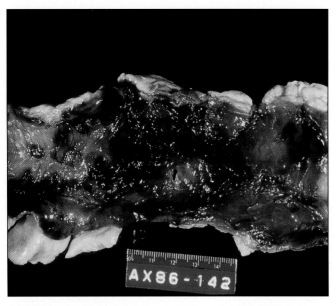

4.9 Necrotizing tracheobronchitis. Note the extensive damage to the mucosa. Cast formation and airway obstruction is very common in this process.

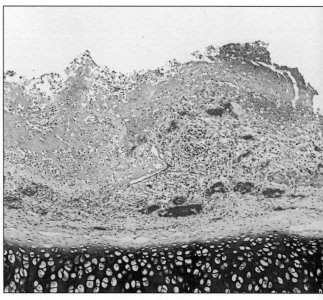

4.10 Mucosal and submucosal injury to the trachea in a patient affected with inhalation injury and respiratory distress syndrome (hematoxylin and eosin, ×200).

SIGNS AND SYMPTOMS OF INHALATION INJURY

4.11 Injury to second-generation bronchi. Note the erosion of the mucosa and the inflammatory response in the mucosa and submucosa (hematoxylin and eosin, ×200).

Signs and symptoms of inhalation injury
• Lacrimation and conjunctivitis
• Severe brassy cough
• Carbonaceous sputum
• Hoarseness
• Shortness of breath
• Wheezing
• Facial burns
• Singed nasal vibrissae
• Stridor
• Bronchorrhea
• Dyspnea
• Anxiety
• Disorientation
• Obtundation
• Coma

4.12 Signs and symptoms of possible inhalation injury. Most patients will present with some combination of the signs and symptoms listed.

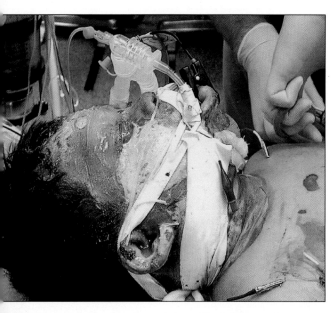

4.13 Patient 24h after burn injury. Facial burns increase the likelihood of inhalation injury to the larynx. Intubation is recommended until bronchoscopic examination of larynx function can be performed.

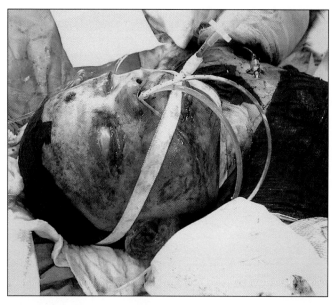

4.14 Same patient as shown in Figure 4.13 at 72h after the burn. Note the marked decrease in facial swelling. The patient had a leak around the endotracheal tube. Larynx function was normal and the patient was extubated.

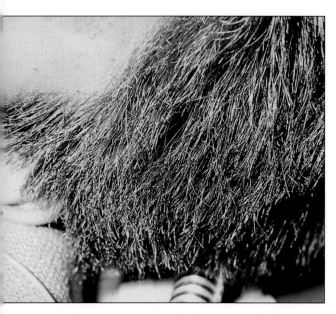

4.15 Singed hair increases the likelihood of inhalation injury. Injury is completely dependent on duration of exposure.

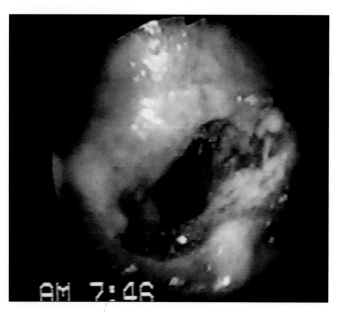

4.16 Singed nasal vibrissae and soot.

GLOTTIC AND SUBGLOTTIC FINDINGS

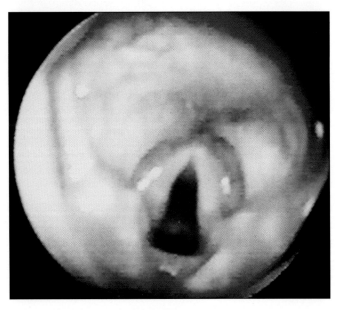

4.17 Larynx venous dilatation.

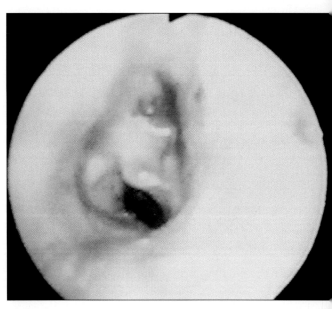

4.18 False cord fibrin cast. Cough reflex and respiratory therapy will resolve this problem.

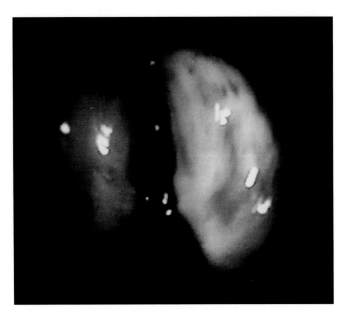

4.19 Carbon on cords is a sign of inhalation injury. Such patients are placed on inhalation injury protocol. Note the molding at the bottom of the cords from transport intubation. The patient was evaluated on arrival and extubated. Molding will resolve spontaneously over time.

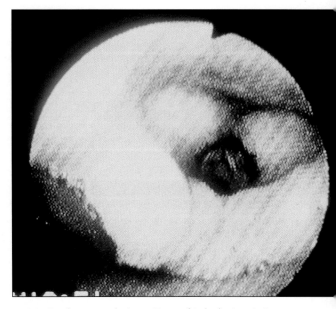

4.20 Carbon cord ring. Sign of inhalation injury.

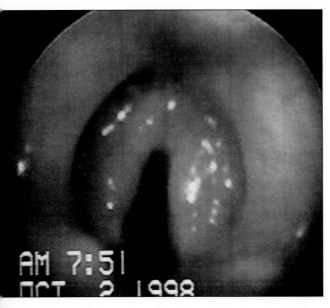

4.21 Edematous larynx with a decrease in opening, but maintaining normal movement. This patient was not intubated except during operative procedures.

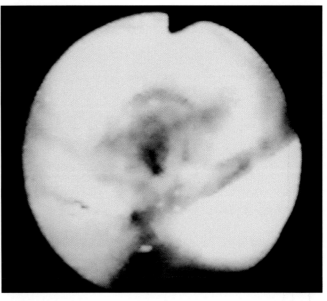

4.22 Burned larynx at 24h. The entire mucosal layer is loose and sloughing. The patient had a good cough reflex and remained extubated.

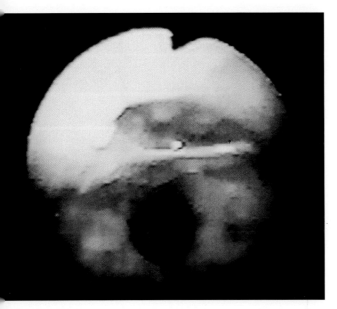

4.23 Burned larynx at 24 hours (close up of 4.22). The entire mucosal layer is loose and sloughing at the epiglottis.

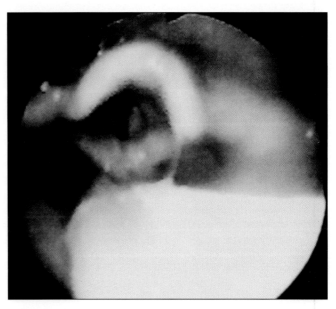

4.24 Burned larynx at 48h. The gray corniculate and cuneiform surfaces are necrotic tissue. The patient was spontaneously ventilating with good cough and was not intubated.

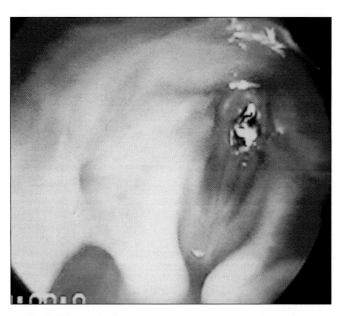

4.25 False cord edema. Larynx view at exhalation. Edema of the corniculates did not restrict ventilation.

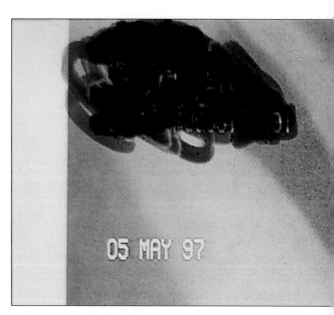

4.26 Corniculate dislocation. Patient presented with hoarseness and quiet voice. Early reduction of the underlying arytenoid/corniculate cartilages is the preferred treatment in these cases.

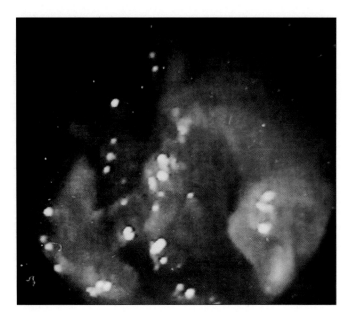

4.27 Subglottic carbon clot. It acted as a ball valve occluding almost the entire trachea. Vigorous saline lavage and suctioning opened the upper bronchial tree.

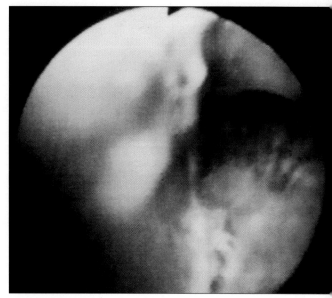

4.28 Subglottic carbon must be cleared by vigorous pulmonary therapy.

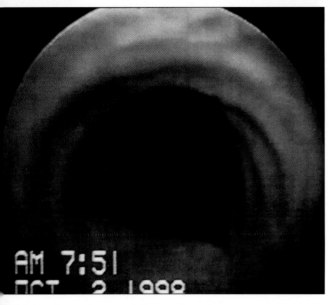

4.29 Early erythema of the trachea. It may progress to tracheal mucosal cast formation and sloughing.

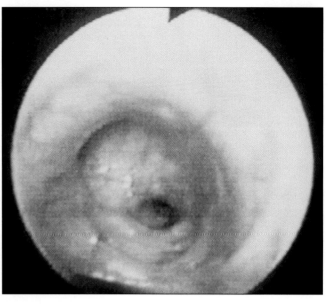

4.30 Bronchial erythema. These lesions may be hemorrhagic and friable.

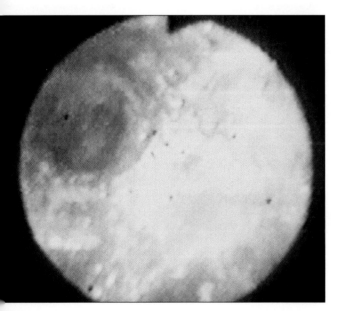

4.31 Necrotizing tracheal bronchitis. The solid eschar formation alternates with loose casts that can occlude the airway. This process continues until a solid scar forms or death occurs.

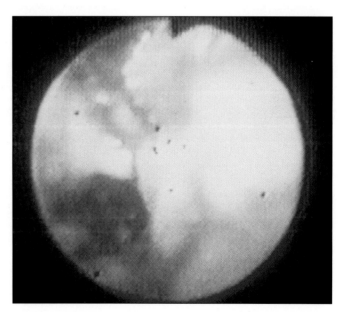

4.32 Total bronchial tree sloughing, causing plugging of bronchial orifices and decreased ventilation. Only vigilant bronchial lavage and suctioning, and bronchial brushing daily or twice a day may maintain these patients until scar tissue is formed.

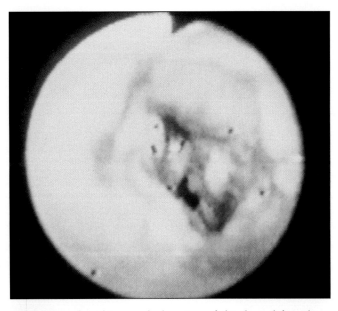

4.33 Cast sloughing and plugging of third- and fourth-generation bronchioles.

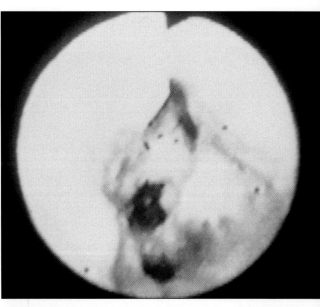

4.34 Cast sloughing in fourth-generation bronchioles.

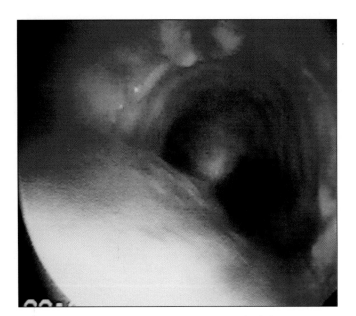

4.35 Tracheal cast formation at the level of the carina tracheae. Severe inhalation injury.

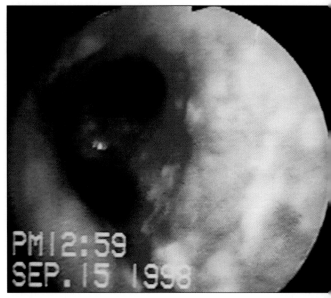

4.36 Tracheal hemorrhage with cast formation 72–96h after injury. Severe inhalation injury.

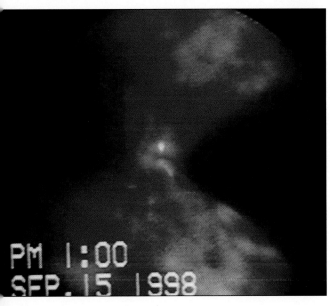

4.37 Tracheal–bronchial hemorrhage with cast formation at the carina tracheae. Severe inhalation injury.

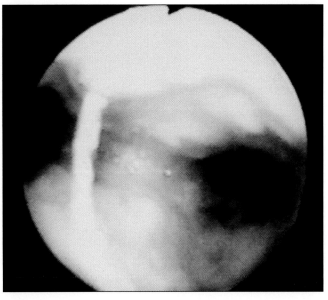

4.38 Cast formation at the carina tracheae. The process is stable at this point until the entire surface sloughs. With a good cough, the patient may clear this him/herself. Severe inhalation injury.

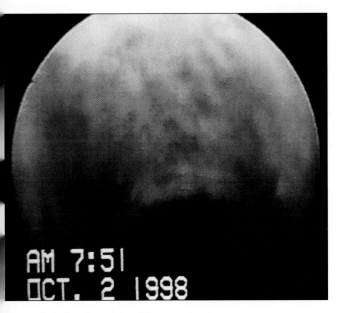

4.39 Subglottic tracheal hemorrhagic spots.

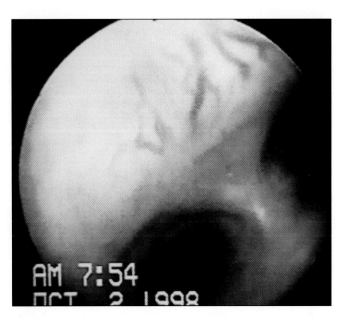

4.40 Classic bronchial vessel engorgement occurs within 12h of inhalation injury and remains for the patient's life time.

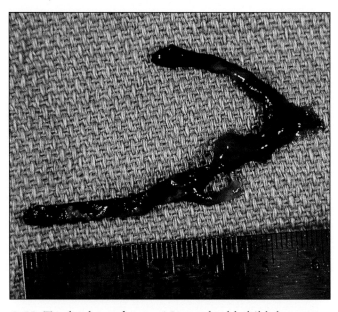

4.41 Tracheal cast from a 15-month-old child that was occluding 75–80% of the airway at the carina tracheae.

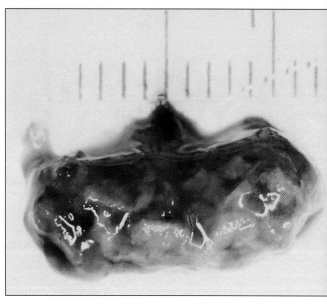

4.42 Tracheal cast.

RESPIRATORY DISTRESS SYNDROME

Etiology of respiratory distress syndrome

- Aspiration
- Central nervous system disease
- Congestive heart failure
- Disseminated intravascular coagulation
- Drug overdose
- Fat or air emboli
- Inhalation injury
- Immunologic reactions
- Massive blood transfusions
- Nonthoracic trauma
- Oxygen toxicity
- Shock
- Thoracic trauma
- Uremia

4.43 Etiology of the respiratory distress syndrome.

Major pathologic or structural changes associated with respiratory distress syndrome

- Interstitial and intra-alveolar edema and hemorrhage
- Intra-alveolar hyaline membrane
- Pulmonary surfactant deficiency or abnormality
- Atelectasis

4.44 Major pathologic/structural changes with respiratory distress syndrome.

Clinical manifestations associated with respiratory distress syndrome

- Increased respiratory rate
- Increased heart rate, cardiac output, and blood pressure
- Pulmonary functions studies:
  Decreased vital capacity
  Decreased residual volume
  Decreased functional residual capacity
  Decreased total lung capacity
  Decreased tidal volume

4.45 Clinical manifestations of respiratory distress syndrome.

Arterial blood gases associated with respiratory distress syndrome

- Early stages
arterial oxygen tension	decreased
arterial carbon dioxide tension	normal or decreased
bicarbonate	normal or decreased
pH	normal or increased

- Advanced stages
arterial oxygen tension	decreased
arterial carbon dioxide tension	increased
bicarbonate	increased
pH	decreased

- Cyanosis
- Chest radiograph findings: increased opacity
- Intercostal retractions
- Chest assessment findings: bronchial breath sounds

4.46 Arterial blood gases associated with respiratory distress syndrome.

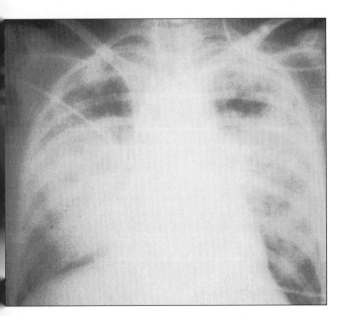

4.47 Chest radiograph showing extensive bilateral alveolar infiltrates.

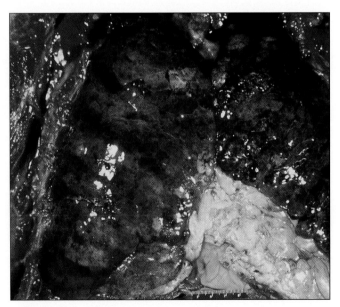

4.48 Gross macroscopic aspect of the lungs in a patient affected by respiratory distress syndrome. Note that the lungs appear consolidated.

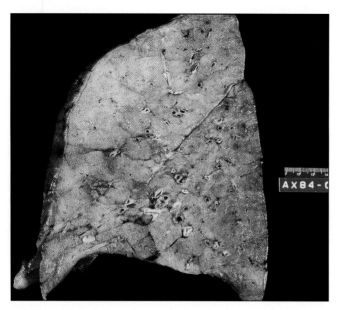

4.49 The infiltrate that occupies the alveoli and the loss of surfactant properties are mainly responsible for the changes to the physiologic properties of the lungs that occur in respiratory distress syndrome. Note that the lung appears solid at cut.

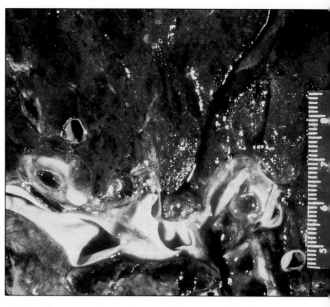

4.50 Close-up view of consolidation of the lung.

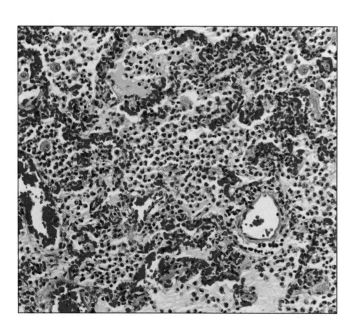

4.51 Early stages of respiratory distress syndrome. Acute and chronic inflammatory infiltrates and hyaline membrane formation occupying the alveoli (hematoxylin and eosin, ×200).

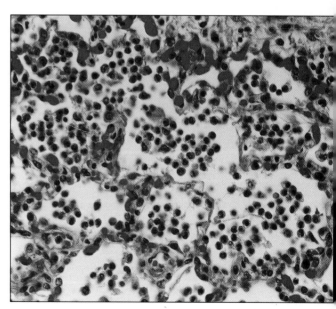

4.52 Pneumocytes types I and II are damaged and replaced by inflammatory cells. Close-up view (hematoxylin and eosin, ×400).

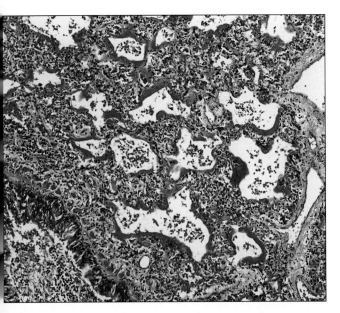

4.53 Late changes of respiratory distress syndrome. Chronic inflammatory infiltrate and collagen deposition to the interstice (hematoxylin and eosin, ×50).

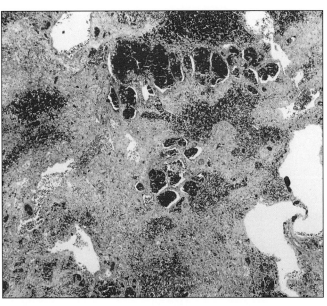

4.54 End-stage of respiratory distress syndrome. Normal architecture has been lost and replaced by scar tissue (trichromic, ×40).

Strategy for managing respiratory distress syndrome

- Humidified gas for spontaneous or artificial ventilation
- Artificial airway for bronchial toilet if secretions are unmanageable
- Increase Functional residual capacity (using positive end-expiratory pressure) to reduce toxic fractional inspired oxygen
- Add mechanical ventilation if work of breathing is excessive
- Adjust tidal volume and positive end-expiratory pressure according to arterial oxygen tension, fractional inspired oxygen, and peak inspiratory pressure
- Avoid neuromuscular blockers if possible
- Consider specialized measures (extracorporeal membrane oxygenation, permissive hypercapnia) to improve gas exchange and oxygen delivery while reducing pulmonary trauma

4.55 Strategies for managing respiratory distress syndrome.

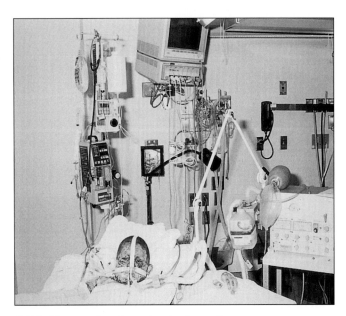

4.56 Conventional mechanical ventilator support. Patients are often managed with the conventional mechanical ventilator in pressure control mode. The key to successful management is to limit the plateau pressure and avoid high fractional inspired oxygen whenever possible.

EARLY COMPLICATIONS

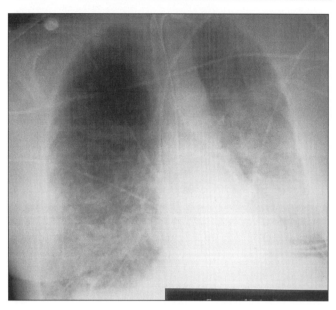

4.57 Chest radiograph showing bilateral pneumonia in a patient affected by inhalation injury. Lobar consolidation frequently develops in patients with extensive *Pseudomonas* infections.

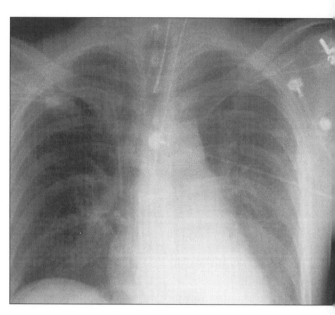

4.58 Chest radiograph. Pneumothorax develops when air escapes into the pleural cavity, allowing the underlying lung to collapse. Breath sounds are decreased on the affected side and oxygenation worsens. Pneumothorax must be suspected in patients treated with high airway pressure. Pneumomediastinum, pneumoperitoneum, and subcutaneous emphysema can also be encountered.

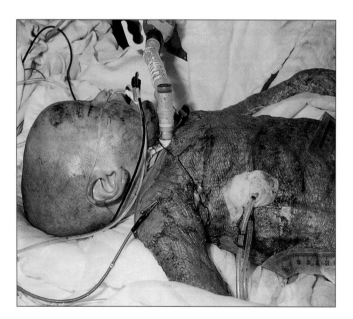

4.59 A child with a right-sided pneumothorax treated with a chest tube.

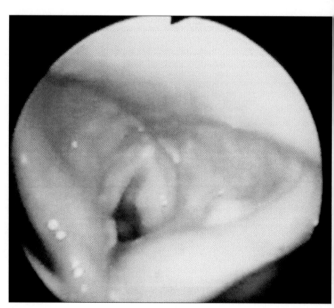

4.60 Postintubation polyp/indentation of right cord. These pathologic findings resolve spontaneously without intervention.

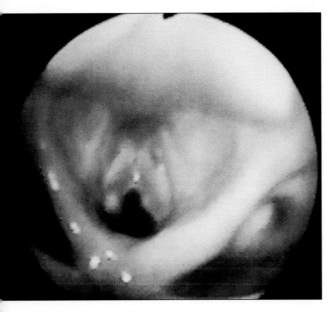

4.61 Cord polyp from intubation.

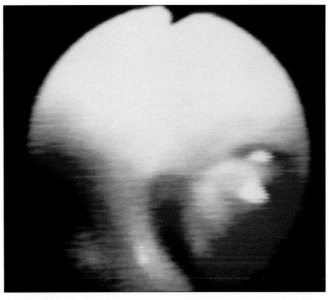

4.62 Bronchial polyp. These types of polyps usually resolve if related to inhalation injury.

LATE COMPLICATIONS

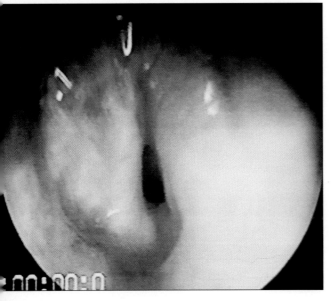

4.63 Glottic stenosis 1 year after heat injury to the glottis. This severe injury required tracheostomy.

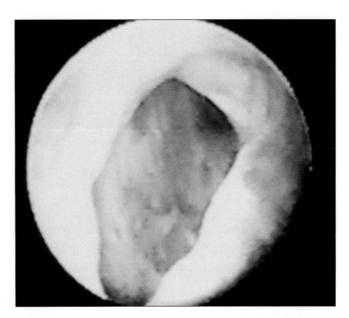

4.64 Classic subglottic tracheal stenosis from inhalation injury, which is below the endotracheal tube cuff level.

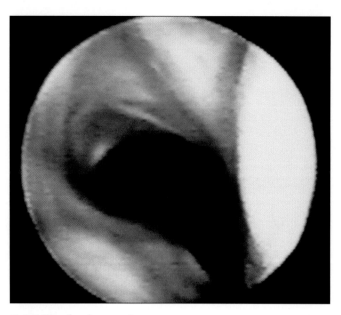

4.65 Tracheal stenosis.

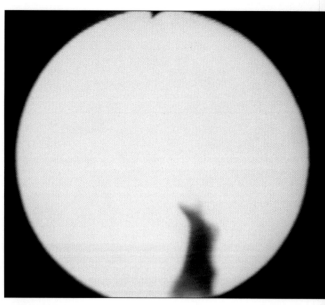

4.66 Severe tracheal stenosis. There is near total occlusion of the trachea.

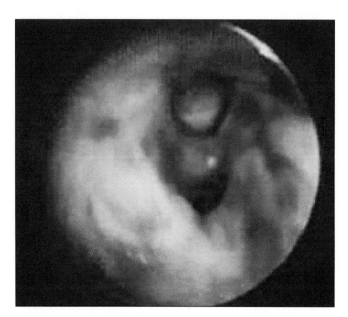

4.67 Tracheal esophageal fistula 1 year after burn injury. The patient is at risk of fatal aspiration.

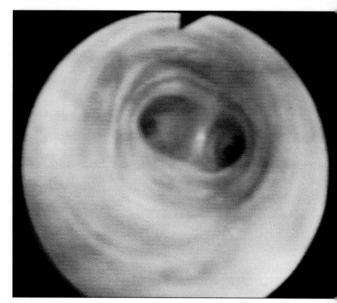

4.68 Tracheal scarring with loss of tracheal rings at the carina tracheae 5 years after burn injury. There is a patient history of 2 months on a ventilator.

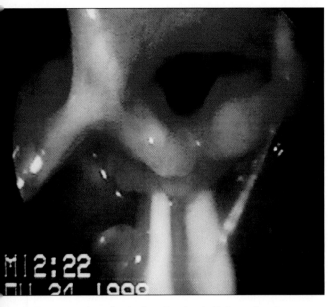

4.69 Laryngeal malacia (expiration). It is a classic postintubation problem in children.

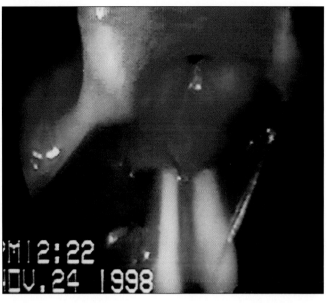

4.70 Laryngeal malacia (inspiration). It can cause severe respiratory compromise and the need for reintubation. In this particular patient, reintubation was required.

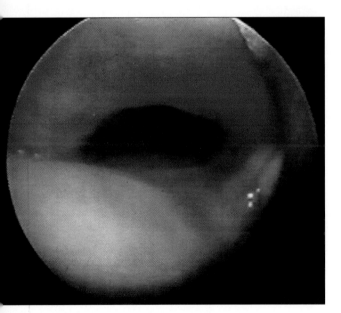

4.71 Tracheal malacia during expiration.

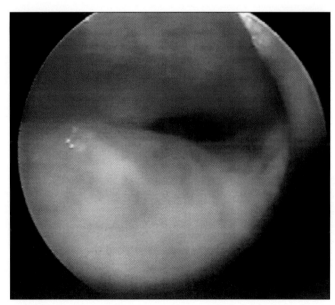

4.72 Tracheal malacia during inspiration. Note the collapse of the trachea due to the lack of cartilage rings.

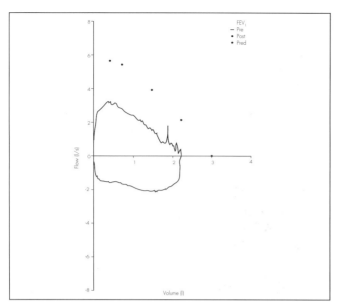

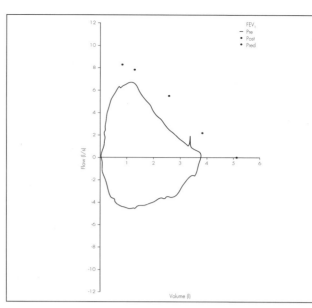

4.73 Obstructive respiratory disease after respiratory distress syndrome. An example of a flow–volume loop from a patient with obstructive lung disease. Patients have a concave configuration of the flow–volume loop, along with a decreased forced vital capacity (FCV), forced expiratory volume in 1s (FEV_1), and forced expiratory flow rate between 25–75% (FEF_{25-75}).

4.74 Restrictive respiratory disease after respiratory distress syndrome. Example of the flow–volume loop from a patient with a purely restrictive disease pattern. They show a convex configuration and a decreased vital capacity, total lung volume, and residual volume (RV). FEV_1, forced expiratory volume in 1s.

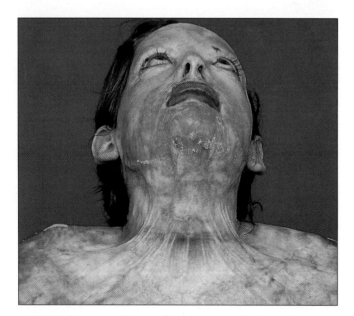

4.75 Tight circumferential scarring can lead to decreased lung function with a restrictive disease component. Chest releases in the late postburn period have shown no significant improvement in lung function, but the patients state that breathing is improved.

RESPIRATORY THERAPY

Inhalation injury protocol

- Titrate high-flow humidified oxygen to maintain arterial oxygen saturation >90%
- Cough, deep breathing exercises every 2h
- Turn patient from one side to the other every 2h
- Chest physiology every 4h
- Nebulize 3ml N-acetylcystine 20% solution every 4h for 7 days
- Nebulize 5000 units of heparin with 3ml of normal saline every 4h for 7 days
- Nasotracheal suctioning as needed
- Early ambulation
- Sputum cultures Monday, Wednesday, and Friday
- Pulmonary function studies before discharge and at scheduled outpatient visits
- Patient/parent education regarding disease process

4.76 Inhalation injury protocol. All patients with positive findings at bronchoscopy or with a positive history of such injury should be placed in this protocol.

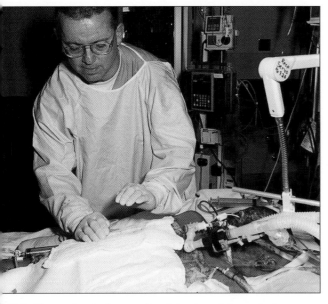

4.77 Chest physiotherapy/positioning. Manual chest physiotherapy and proper positioning for postural drainage aids in the removal of secretions/cast from the airway.

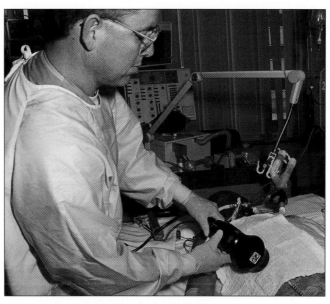

4.78 Percussion/vibrations. The use of a hand-held percussion device can be useful for secretion clearance. (Care must be used to not destroy skin grafts.)

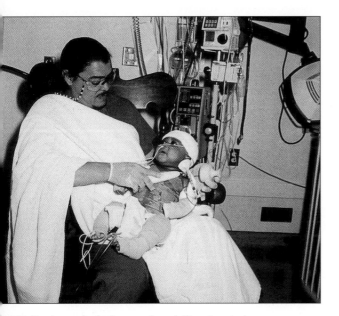

4.79 Early ambulation and mobilization is important to aid in secretion removal, to prevent atelectasis and pneumonia, and to improve oxygenation.

American College of Chest Physicians Consensus Conference on Mechanical Ventilation

- The clinician should choose a ventilator mode that has been shown to be capable of supporting oxygenation/ventilation in patients with adult respiratory distress syndrome and that the clinician has experience in using

- An acceptable oxygen saturation should be targeted

- When plateau pressure equals or exceeds $35cmH_2O$, the tidal volume should be decreased (to as low as 5ml/kg, and lower, if necessary); in conditions where chest wall compliance is low, plateau pressures somewhat greater than $35cmH_2O$ may be acceptable

- To limit plateau pressures, permissive hypercapnia should be considered, unless other contraindications exist that demand a more normal carbon dioxide tension (PCO_2) and pH

- Positive end-expiratory pressure (PEEP) is useful in supporting oxygenation. The level of PEEP required should be established by empiric trials and re-evaluated on a regular basis

- Large tidal volumes (12–15ml/kg) may be needed to improve oxygenation. Peak flow rates should be adjusted as needed to satisfy the patient's inspiratory demands

- Current opinion is that fractional inspired oxygen (FiO_2) should be kept as low as possible. However, to maintain oxygenation at lower FiO_2's, higher alveolar pressures may be needed. When both high alveolar pressures and high FiO_2's are required to maintain oxygenation, it is reasonable to accept an arterial oxygen saturation slightly less than 90%

- When oxygenation is inadequate, sedation, paralysis, and position changes are possible corrective measures. Other factors in oxygen delivery, such as cardiac output and hemoglobin, should also be considered

4.80 The American College of Chest Physicians Consensus Conference on Mechanical Ventilation gives an overview of the recommended use of mechanical ventilation. With permission from *Chest* 1993; 104:1833–59.

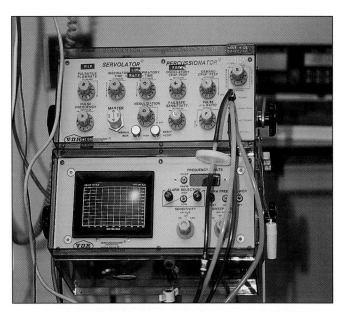

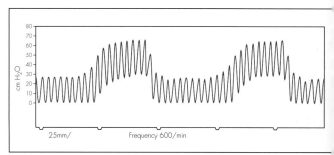

4.82 Volumetric diffusive respiration wave form. The waveform illustrates the percussive nature of this mode of ventilation. Note the percussive nature on inspiration and expiration. This aids in the removal of fibrin casts and secretions.

4.81 Volumetric diffusive respiration ventilator. This mode of ventilation is referred to as high-frequency percussive ventilation. It has been shown to decrease barotrauma, decrease the incidence of pneumonia, and improve oxygenation. This mode of ventilation can be thought of as pressure control with high-frequency percussive capabilities.

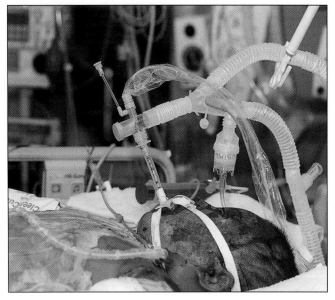

4.83 Securing endotracheal tubes in burn patients can present a challenge. Our technique involves securing the tube with one strap under the ears and the other strap over the ears.

CHAPTER 5
WOUND CARE

Juan P. Barret, MD and John P. Heggers, PhD

BURN WOUND HEALING

Burn wound healing	
First-degree burns	Epidermis only damaged Area initially erythematous due to vasodilatation Desquamation in 7 days with complete scarless healing
Second-degree burns	Epidermis and various degrees of dermis destroyed Healing occurs through migration to the surface, of epithelial cells that survive in deeper portions of hair follicles as well as in sweat and sebaceous glands Almost scarless in superficial injuries, although hypertrophic scarring may occur in deeper injuries
Third-degree burns	Involves necrosis of the entire thickness of the skin Leaves minor chances for healing except for very small wounds, which may heal by contraction and epithelization

5.1 Principles of healing in different burn wounds.

Considerations in burn wound healing
• Second-degree burns that heal within 3 weeks are unlikely to leave scars
• Injury to deep structures and prolonged inflammatory processes in the wound enhance hypertrophic scarring
• Zone of stasis may convert to necrosis in second-degree burns
• Deep second-degree burns should be treated as full thickness or third-degree burns, with excision and autografting

5.2 An assessment as to whether the wound will heal within 3 weeks is of paramount importance in order to consider topical treatment or excision and autografting. The latter is believed to shorten the inflammatory process and render better scars than prolonged wound healing.

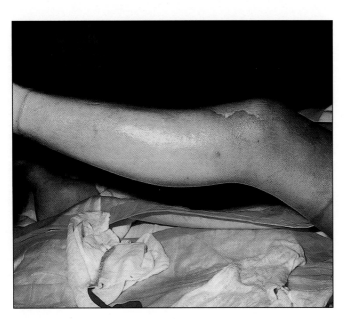

5.3 Superficial second-degree burn to the lower extremities. Treatment with silver sulfadiazine.

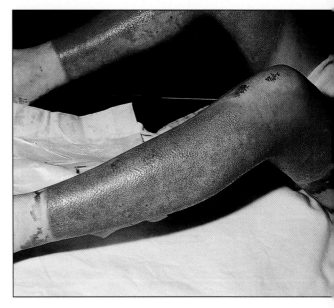

5.4 Same patient as shown in Figure 5.3, 4 days later. Note that epithelial regeneration has started from the hair follicles and sweat glands.

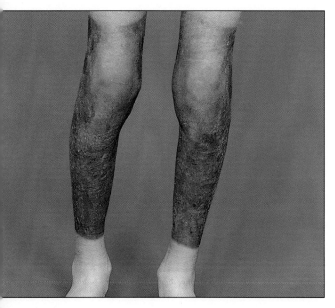

5.5 Same patient as shown in Figure 5.3, 2 months after the injury. Vasodilatation and hyperpigmentation is present.

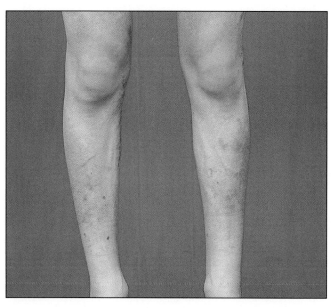

5.6 Same patient as shown in Figure 5.3, 18 months after the injury. Scarring and sequelae are minimal.

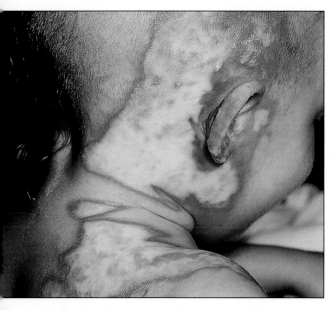

5.7 Superficial and deep second-degree scald burns to the head, face, and shoulder. Treatment is with silver sulfadiazine.

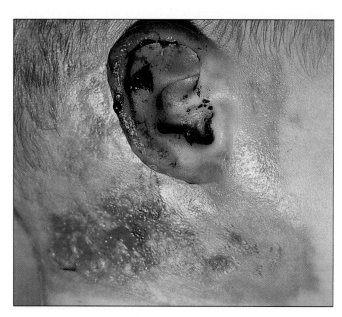

5.8 Same patient as shown in in Figure 5.7, 12 days after the injury. Note that most of the injury is healed.

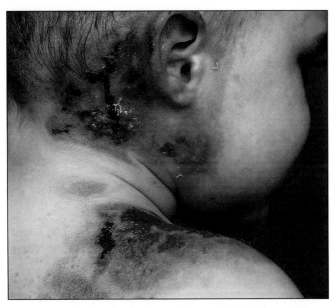

5.9 Same patient as shown in Figure 5.7, 26 days after the injury. Deep second-degree wounds are still healing. Note that all superficial second-degree burns are healed and maturing.

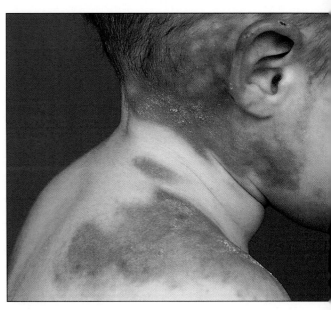

5.10 Same patient as shown in Figure 5.7, 2 months after the injury. All wounds are healed. Vasodilatation is present.

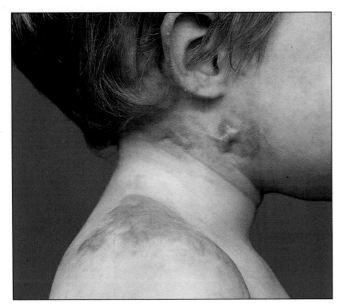

5.11 Same patient as shown in Figure 5.7, 6 months after the injury. The patient has hypertrophic scarring in areas that took longer than 3 weeks to heal.

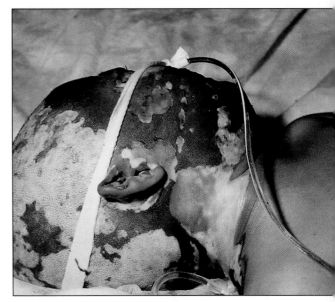

5.12 Deep-second degree and third-degree flame burns to the head.

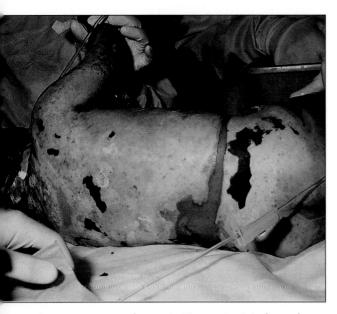

5.13 Same patient as shown in Figure 5.12 in lateral decubitus position, showing third-degree burns to the back.

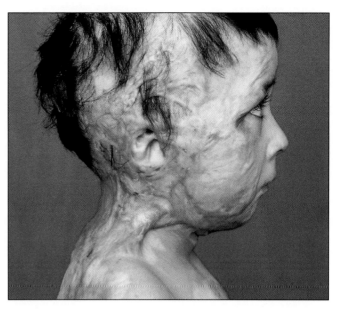

5.14 Same patient as shown in Figure 5.12, 9 months after the injury. All burns were treated with excision and autografting. Note the various degrees of alopecia and complete absence of the right ear.

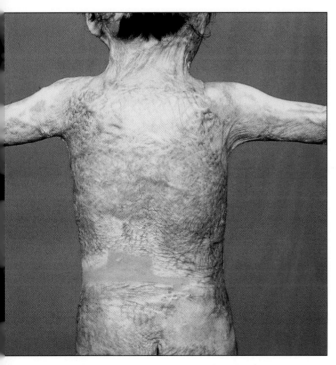

5.15 Same patient as shown in Figure 5.12. Burns to the back were treated also with excision and autografting. Although scarring does occur after autografting, the degree of hypertrophic scarring and functional impairment is believed to be less than with spontaneous healing.

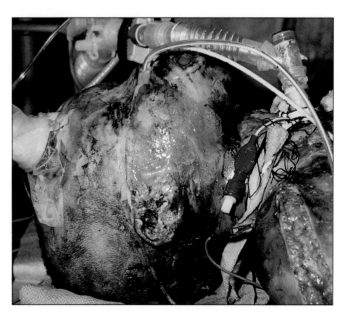

5.16 Fourth-degree burns to the face in a 98% total body surface area full thickness injury. All layers of the skin and different layers of deep tissues are destroyed.

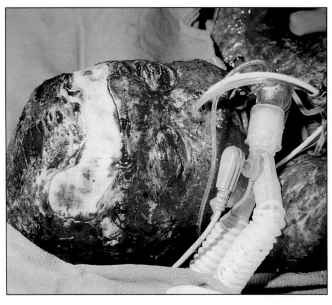

5.17 Same patient as shown in Figure 5.16, 3 weeks after the injury, treated with immediate excision and homografting. Note the exposed frontal bone.

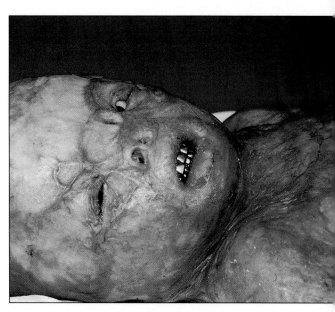

5.18 Same patient as shown in Figure 5.16, 6 months after the injury. Wounds were closed with cultured epithelial cells. Hypertrophic scarring with this technique is significant.

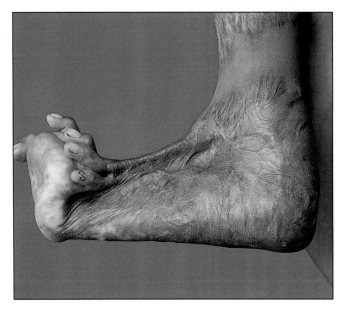

5.19 Neglected deep injuries result in important functional impairment if left untreated. Spontaneous wound healing tends to contract to diminish the gap between normal tissues.

MANAGEMENT OF PATIENTS

Factors to consider regarding inpatient versus outpatient management

- Age: patients between 5 and 34 years of age have the most favorable outcomes
- Extent of the injury: follow ABA criteria for referral and admission to a burn center
- Depth of the burn
- Premorbid diseases
- Comorbid disorders
  Associated trauma
  Distribution of a burn
  Injuring agent
  Social circumstances
- Pain control
- Difficulty in providing wound care

5.20 Different factors need to be assessed in order to decide whether a patient can be treated either as an outpatient or should be admitted to the burn center. Patients with extensive burns can be treated as outpatients once resuscitation has been completed. An individual approach to the latter is essential, with treatment tailored to each patient. ABA, American Burn Association.

Purposes of a dressing

- To absorb draining fluids
- To provide protection and isolation of a wound from the environment
- To decrease wound pain

5.21 Dogmatic recommendations cannot be made for dressing wounds. If the dressing does not serve any of these three purposes, it may not be needed.

Burn wound dressings available

- Nonmedicinal white petrolatum-impregnated fine mesh (Adaptic)
- Fine mesh absorbent gauze impregnated with 3% bismuth tribromophenate (Xeroform)
- Bacitracin ointment
- Mupirocin ointment
- Polymyxin B ointment
- Nystatin ointment
- Silver sulfadiazine
- Cerium nitrate sulfadiazine
- Mafenide
- 0.5% Silver nitrate solution
- 0.025% Sodium hypochlorite solution
- Nitrofurazone
- Chlorhexidine
- Povidone–iodine
- Combination therapy
- Pig skin
- Synthetic wound dressings (Biobrane, OpSite, Mepitel, etc.)

5.22 Different types of dressings and techniques are available for wound care. They range from leaving the wound exposed, to use of synthetic materials. The breadth of wound care is as wide as the physician's imagination.

Wound care of burn injuries

First-degree burns and very superficial second-degree burns	Nonmedicinal white petrolatum-impregnated fine mesh and skin lotions; no dressing required
Second-degree burns	Silver sulfadiazine Mafenide in infected burns Calcium alginate Acticoat Homografts (large, life-threatening, second-degree burns) Biobrane, OpSite, Trancyte, Mepitel, pig skin Excision and autografting versus skin substitutes in deep second-degree burns
Third-degree burns	Excision and autografting versus skin substitutes Cerium nitrate sulfadiazine

5.23 General recommendations for burn wound care.

Wound care of skin auto/homografts

- Fine mesh gauze impregnated with polymyxin B and Mycostatin
- Polysporin
- Bactroban
- Nitrofurazone
- Biobrane
- Mepitel
- Silver nitrate and mafenide solutions in infected grafts
- Half per cent Dakin's solution (sodium hypochlorite)
- Wet–wet and wet–dry dressing changes
- Topical nystatin powder

5.24 Different dressings and topical materials are available for graft care. The most important principle is to minimize trauma and shearing forces while engrafting is taking place.

5. WOUND CARE

Wound care for donor sites
• Petrolatum-impregnated fine mesh gauze
• Fine mesh gauze impregnated with scarlet red
• Silver sulfadiazine
• Biobrane
• OpSite
• Mepitel
• Acticoat

5.25 Keeping a moist, clean environment is the most crucial factor for regrowth of keratinocytes in donor sites.

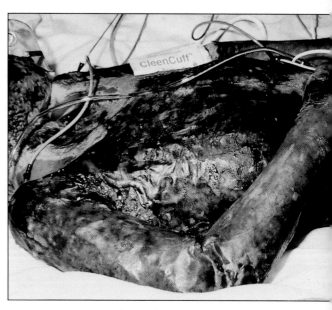

5.26 Exposure method of wound care with tannic acid in a 12-year-old patient affected by an 85% total body surface area full thickness burn. With this treatment, the burn eschar desiccates and eventually separates by the action of bacterial collagenases. A high incidence of sepsis, mortality, and conversion to full thickness injuries in survivors is common with this technique.

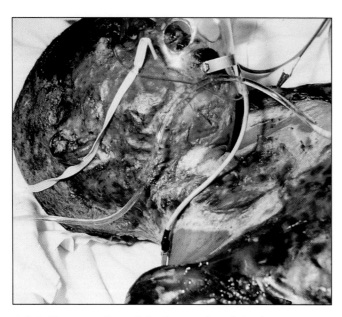

5.27 Close-up view of the face and neck in the same patient as shown in Figure 5.26.

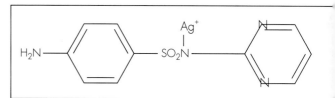

5.28 Silver sulfadiazine formula. Note the ion Ag and the sulfanilamide part.

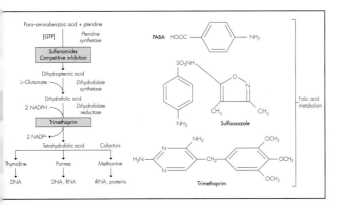

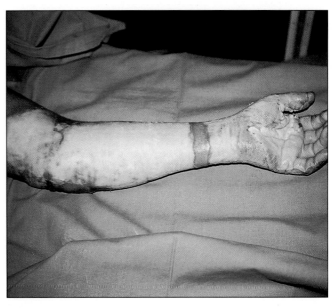

5.29 Mechanism of action for silver sulfadiazine is twofold. First, the mechanism relies on the oligodynamic effect of the metallic ion Ag, which at 1 part per million effectively interferes with protein synthesis. The sulfanilamide interferes with intermediary metabolism of microorganisms that can synthesize para-aminobenzoate (PABA) for folate production or for growth. GTP, guanosine triphosphate; NADP, nicotinamide adenine dinucleotide phosphate; NADPH, reduced form of NADP; tRNA, transfer RNA.

5.30 Typical appearance of a superficial and a deep second-degree burn after 4 days of treatment with silver sulfadiazine. Note the pseudo-eschar that this treatment typically produces in burn wounds.

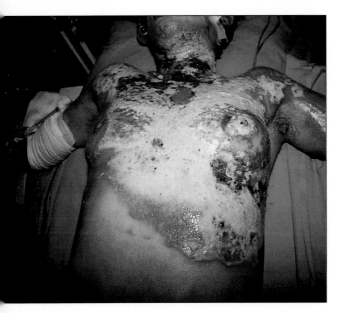

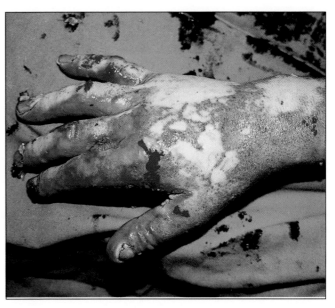

5.31 Deep second-degree burns treated for 10 days with silver sulfadiazine. Note that the edges are regenerating. Pseudo-eschar challenges the evaluation of the wounds. Foul smell, discoloration, surrounding cellulitis, and eschar separation are signs of infection.

5.32 Pseudo-eschar usually separates when the epidermis is regenerating underneath.

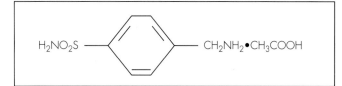

5.33 Mafenide acetate formula (Sulfamylon cream or solution). Mafenide acetate effectively interferes with folic acid metabolism as a competitive inhibitor preventing the conversion of PABA to dihydropteroic acid, consequently inhibiting amino acid synthesis.

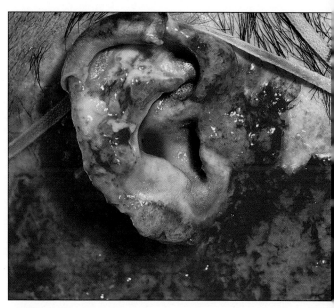

5.34 Mafenide penetrates extremely well into tissues. It is the first choice to treat burns to the ears, because its penetration is excellent. It is also very helpful for the treatment of infected wounds. Disadvantages include pain and metabolic acidosis, especially if large areas are exposed to the agent.

Cerium nitrate–silver sulfadiazine	
Formula	Cerium nitrate: $Ce(NO_3)_36H_2O$ Silver sulfadiazine
Action	Both metals have an oligodynamic effect and interfere with the nucleic acid synthesis of the organism, while the sulfadiazine interferes with intermediary metabolism
Microbiology	Gram-positive: active against staphylococci, streptococci, and enterococci Gram-negative: active against the enterics, along with *Pseudomonas aeruginosa*

5.35 Cerium is a rare-earth metal that has an oligodynamic effect similar to that of silver. It is readily available and has a low toxicity. In combination with silver sulfadiazine, it provides a more efficacious bacteriostasis than achieved individually. It can cause pain on application, and side effects include methemoglobinemia.

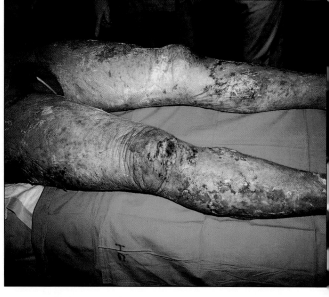

5.36 Full thickness burns to the lower extremities treated with cerium nitrate sulfadiazine. Note that the eschar becomes more rigid and may even calcify. This kind of treatment permits delayed excision of treated areas. On tangential excision, the burn wound feels and behaves similarly to a fresh wound.

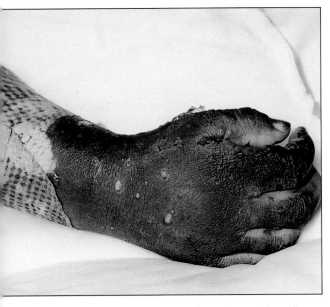

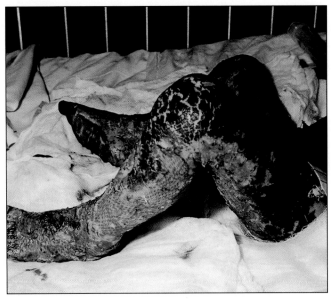

5.37 Silver nitrate treatment on infected wounds. Silver nitrate solution is anti-infective; weak solutions are used germicidally. Silver nitrate should be kept hydrated at all times. If dry, it precipitates, and impairs wound healing.

5.38 Treatment with silver nitrate. Note that it has precipitated and some autografts are melting due to the deleterious effect.

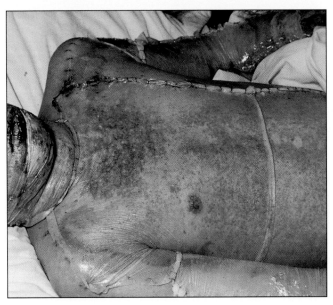

5.39 Superficial and small areas of deep second-degree scald burns before topical treatment: 25% total body surface area.

5.40 Treatment of the same patient as shown in Figure 5.39 with the application of Biobrane. The patient has to be monitored for the development of infection. Advantages of Biobrane are that it is painless and dressing changes are not necessary.

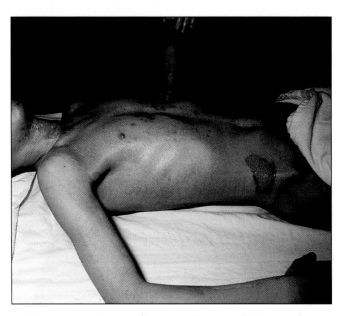

5.41 Same patient as shown in Figure 5.40. Seven days after the injury most of it has closed. Biobrane peels off when the wound has healed underneath.

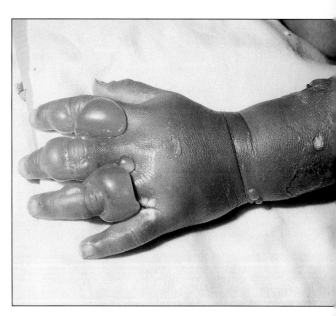

5.42 Superficial second-degree burns to the hand and forearm. Note the swelling and blistering.

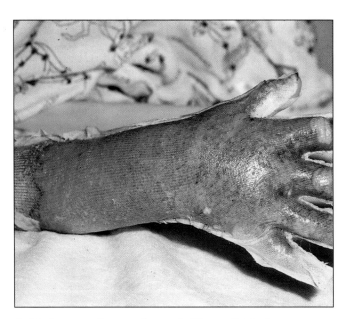

5.43 Same patient as shown in Figure 5.42 after treatment with a Biobrane glove.

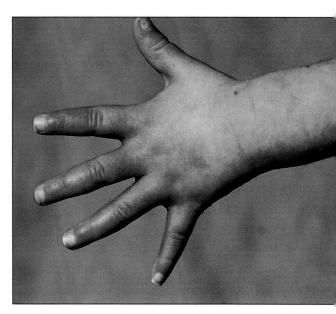

5.44 Same patient as shown in Figure 5.42, 1 month later. Discoloration and hyperemia is minimal.

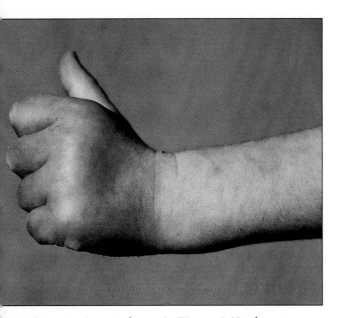

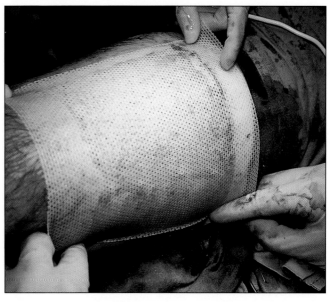

5.45 Same patient as shown in Figure 5.42 after treatment. The patient now has a full range of motion without restrictions or problems of dry skin. Treatment of partial thickness burns in children is extremely effective due to the absence of pain in the recovery phase.

5.46 Mepitel, a silicone mesh that adapts to the wound, is also effective in controlling pain and promotes wound healing. It can be used in partial thickness burns, donor sites, and engrafted areas.

CHAPTER 6

SURGICAL CLOSURE OF THE BURN WOUND

Juan P. Barret, MD

GENERAL PRINCIPLES

Wounds that benefit from excision and grafting
• Burns with indeterminate depth (partial thickness burns with a mixture of superficial and deep second degree) that do not heal within 3 weeks • Deep second-degree burns • Full thickness (third and fourth degree) burns • Infected burns

6.1 Certain deep dermal injuries and full thickness injuries benefit from excision of all dead tissue and autografting. Such treatment results in better function and cosmetic appearance. Indeterminate burns should be assessed to determine whether they will heal within 3 weeks. If not, surgical closure is recommended.

Techniques used in burn surgery
• Primary closure of excised burns and/or donor sites • Amputation • Tangential or laminar excision • Fascial excision • Degloving (avulsion)

6.2 Different techniques are used for wound closure. Tangential excision and autografting with medium thickness split autografts provide the best outcome.

Surgical wound closure in patients with non-life-threatening burns
• Most patients fall into this category • Ample skin graft donor sites are present • Excision and grafting with sheet grafts within a few days after the burn has occurred is the treatment of choice • Permanent wound closure is achieved in one, or occasionally two operative procedures

6.3 Most of the injuries encountered in burn centers are small injuries that are suitable for early excision and sheet autografting.

Early total excision and staged surgical wound closure in burns covering greater than 30% body surface area	
Early total excision	All deep partial and full thickness burns are excised on admission Autografts are taken from areas that are not burned and grafted to the trunk or lower extremities; the rest of the burn is homografted or covered with skin substitutes Patient returns to the operating theater when donor sites are available (usually at weekly intervals) for further autografting until the entire wound is closed
Staged surgical wound closure	Staged excision of unequivocally deep burns at intervals of approximately 7 days Immediate coverage of excised wounds with autografts or skin substitutes First operative procedure within 3–5 days Patients may return in 48h for further excision of deep burns if the new generation of dermal substitutes is used (i.e. Integra)

6.4 Both early total burn wound excision and staged surgical excision have advantages and disadvantages. The goal is to excise all dead tissue before the wound becomes infected.

ANESTHESIA FOR BURN PATIENTS

Techniques of wound closure

- Sheet autografts
- Autografts meshed 1:1, 1.5:1, 2:1, 3:1
- Sandwich technique (homografts overlying widely expanded meshed 4:1 or 6:1 autografts)
- Homografts
- Trancyte
- Biobrane
- AlloDerm
- Integra
- Cultured epidermal autografts

6.5 Techniques for wound closure need to be tailored to individual patient needs.

General principles in burn anesthesia

- Continuous control of the airway
- Intubation under direct bronchoscopy
- Surgeon available in the operating theater for emergent tracheostomy if needed
- Nasotracheal intubation as first choice
- Spontaneous ventilation throughout the operative session
- Full monitoring
- All blood requirements should be in the room before surgery starts
- Anesthetist scrubbed for easy access to all areas

6.6 Experienced burn anesthetists are important members of the burn team. Skills in pediatric and adult burn anesthesia are necessary, along with a thorough knowledge of burn pathophysiology and critical care medicine.

Monitoring during surgery

- Continuous electrocardiography
- Continuous respiratory rate monitoring
- Pulse-oximeter
- Temperature probe
- Foley
- Central line
- Large bore peripheral intravenous catheter (or large bore central line)
- Capnometer
- Arterial line

6.7 Monitoring during surgery.

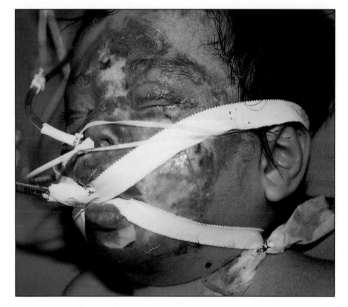

6.8 Tube fixation during surgery is extremely important. When operating on the face, the tube can be wired to the teeth if in the oral position, or tied to the nasal septum if in the nasal position.

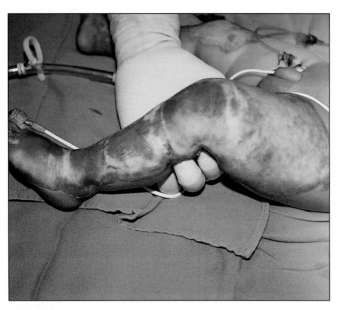

6.9 Foley catheter and temperature probe, arterial lines, and pulse-oximeters are important parts of monitoring.

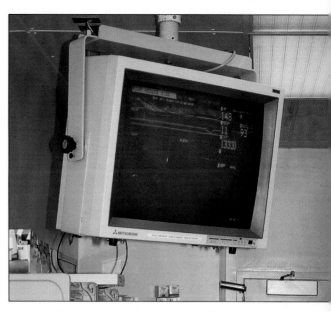

6.10 Ceiling monitors are very useful to control all parameters during burn surgery. They can easily be read by the anesthetist and burn surgeon at any time during the operation.

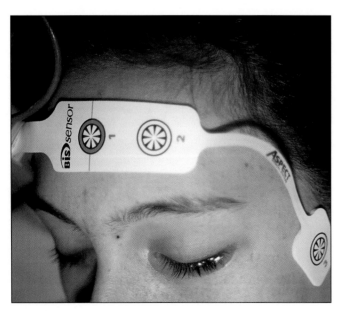

6.11 Electroencephalography probes are an additional method to monitor the level of anesthesia.

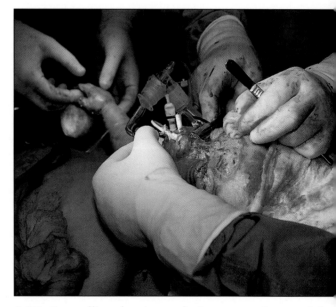

6.12 Controlling the airway during surgery is essential. A scrubbed anesthetist can adjust the tube and reach any part of the patient's body without compromising sterile conditions during surgery.

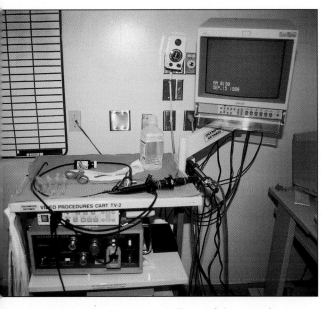

6.13 Bronchoscopes are especially useful to intubate patients and to assess the extent of inhalation injury.

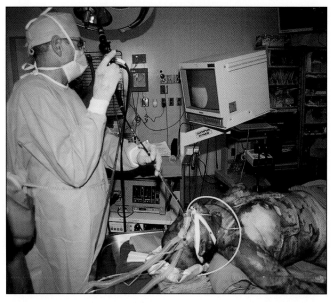

6.14 Nasotracheal intubation is performed under direct vision with the aid of bronchoscopy. A surgeon should be ready to perform a tracheostomy if the airway can not be secured.

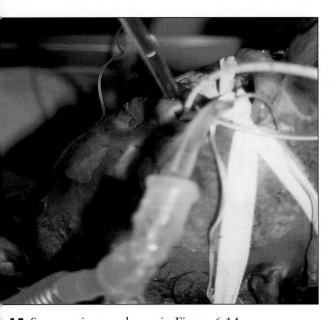

6.15 Same patient as shown in Figure 6.14. Nasotracheal intubation in a severely burned patient. Note that the tube has been introduced into the bronchoscope.

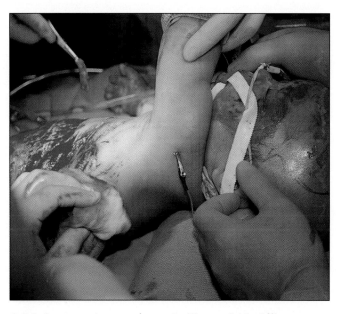

6.16 Same patient as shown in Figure 6.14. Alligator-type electrocardiography probes are very useful in burn surgery. They can be attached to a skin staple and retain good contact during the duration of the operation.

Calculation of expected blood loss	
Less than 24h from injury	0.45ml/cm² burn area
1–3 days since burn injury	0.70ml/cm² burn area
More than 4 days since burn injury	0.90ml/cm² burn area
Infected burn wounds	1.0–1.25ml/cm² burn area

6.17 Blood loss can be extensive during burn surgery. The expected loss of blood must be calculated before surgery so that sufficient quantities can be ordered in advance.

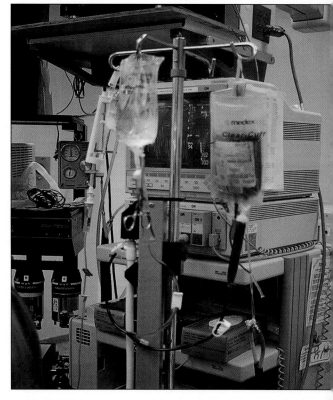

6.18 Fluid warmers help to maintain core temperature at above 37°C.

THE OPERATING ROOM

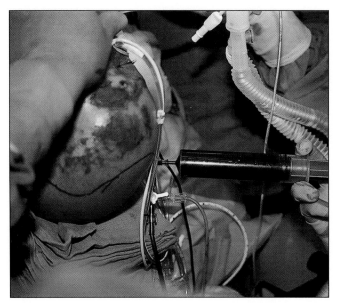

6.19 Same patient as shown in Figure 6.14. Blood pumping is often necessary to ensure that any blood loss is immediately replaced. Hematocrit and other hematologic, blood gas, and blood chemistry parameters should be checked every 20–30min during the operation.

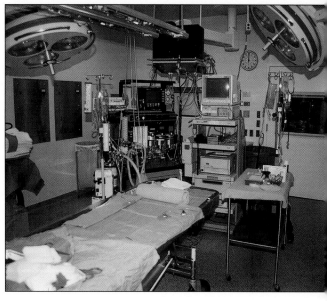

6.20 Typical appearance of the burn operating theater. Large and spacious operating rooms with all equipment ready and available help when performing large excisions.

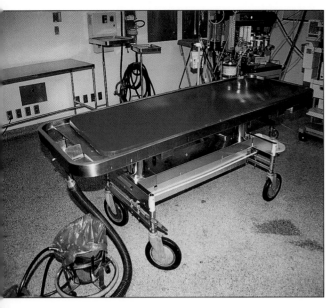

6.21 The burn operating table. This special table helps in performing full body preparation and gaining quick access to any anatomic area of the patient.

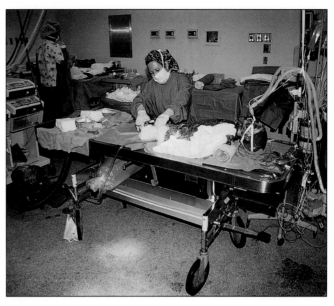

6.22 The burn patient can be prepared with warm running water and Betadine scrubbing. Overhead heaters help to keep the patient warm.

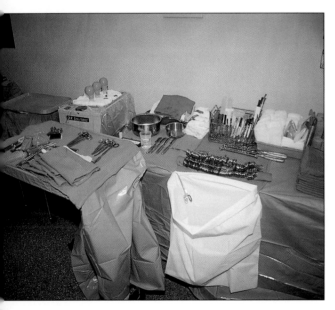

6.23 The whole room has to be prepared before the patient arrives. All instruments, including dermatomes, and skin meshers, dressings, etc., have to be ready for use.

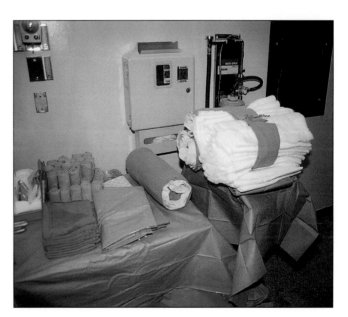

6.24 The burn dressings are ready to apply so that no time is wasted during the operation.

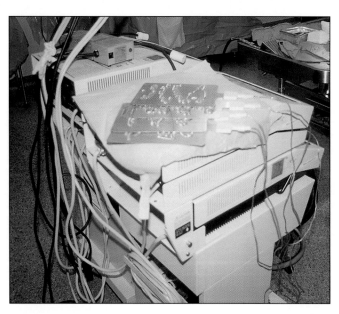

6.25 Bovie plates are very useful during burn surgery. As long as the patient is positioned on the plates, there is good contact and electrocautery can be used safely.

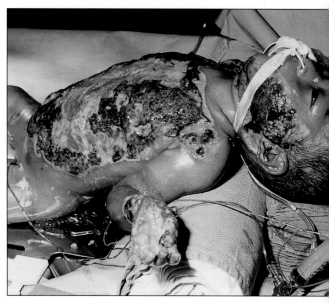

6.26 Patient positioned on Bovie plates. After the full body preparation, the position of the patient on them thereon can be changed during surgery to maintain good contact.

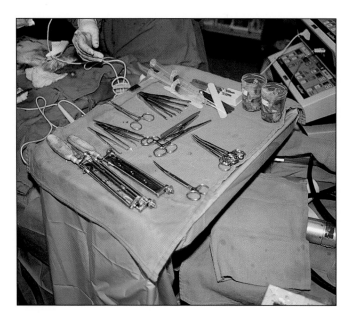

6.27 The Watson dermatome. It can be used for both excision and skin harvesting, although better precision can be achieved with the automatic dermatomes. For smaller areas, the Goulian dermatome can be used.

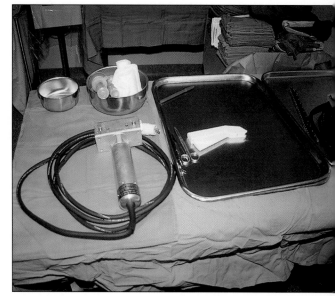

6.28 The Padgett dermatome. Different guards help to harvest skin grafts with different widths. It is very important to insure that all the mobile pieces are well adjusted, so that a full thickness skin harvest does not result.

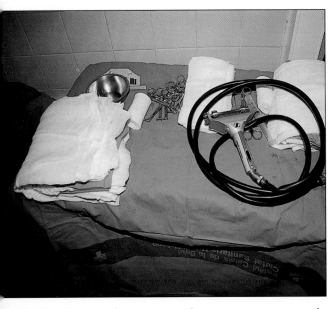

6.29 The Zimmer dermatome. The same comments and precautions as given in the caption to Figure 6.28 apply.

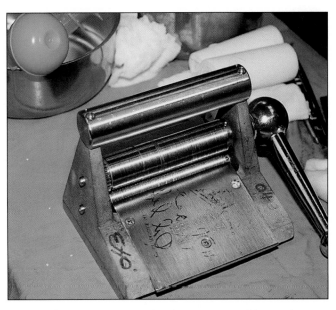

6.30 When tissue expansion is necessary, skin meshers, an example of which is illustrated here, are used. Expansions of 1:1, 1.5:1, 2:1, 3:1, 4:1, 6:1, and 9:1 can be performed with different types of meshers.

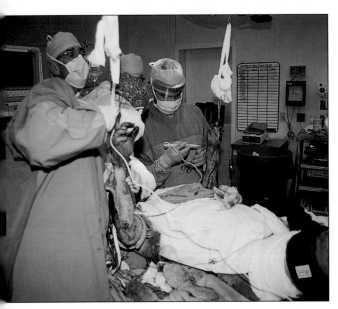

6.31 Ceiling hooks can be utilized to elevate and suspend the limbs while the operation is in progress.

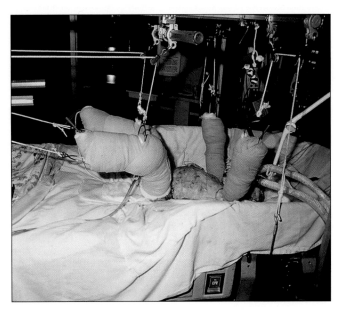

6.32 Under certain circumstances the patient needs to be in skeletal traction.

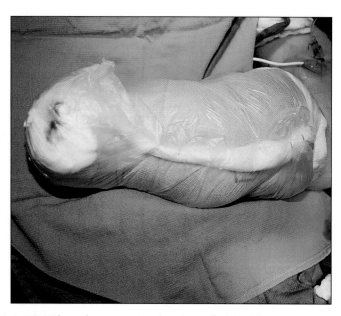

6.33 When the operation has been finished in one anatomic location, dressing the area and wrapping limbs with plastic bags helps to prevent heat and evaporative losses.

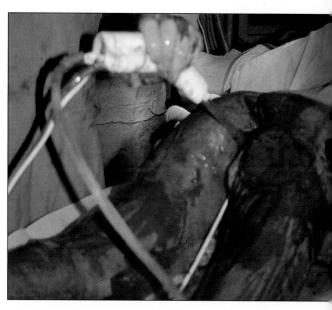

6.34 Jet lavage with pressurized saline, and using antibiotic solutions in infected wounds, helps to decrease the bacterial count after wound debridement.

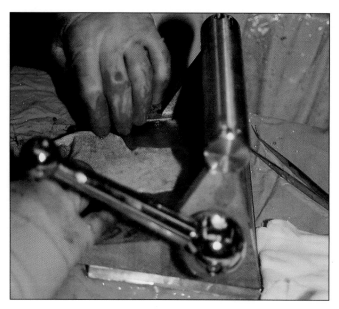

6.35 Meshing technique. The skin autograft is placed on the mesher, with the epidermal side facing the device.

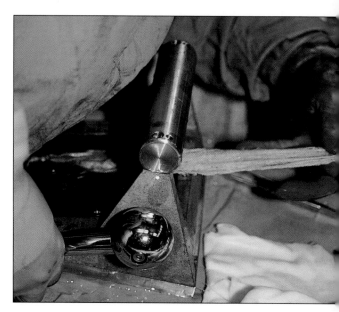

6.36 The skin graft is passed through the mesher with extreme care so that the graft does not roll onto the mesher drum.

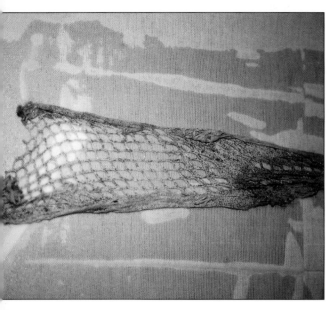

6.37 Finally, the skin graft is placed over wet fine-mesh gauze. The dermal side must be kept moist in order to maintain graft viability.

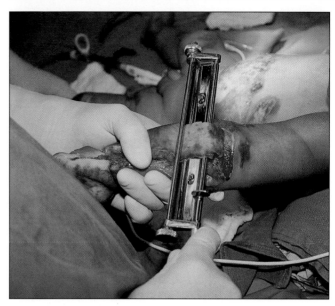

6.38 Tangential excision with the Watson knife. Layers of tissue are excised sequentially until living tissue with punctate bleeding is reached.

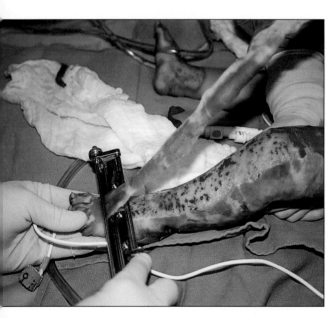

6.39 An assistant maintaining traction on the eschar is very helpful in performing excision when deep tissues are to be reached. If deep dermis is to be spared, traction should be avoided.

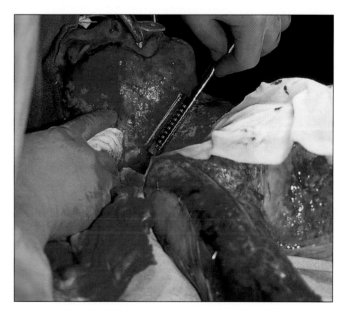

6.40 The Goulian knife is often utilized in performing excisions on the hands and face. It is supplied with different guards for different depths.

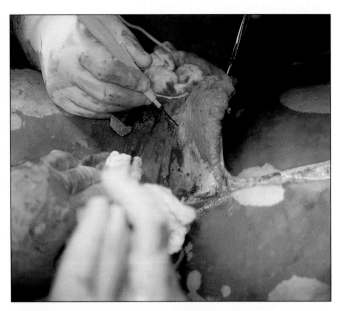

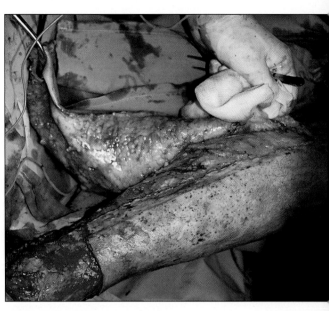

6.41 Fascial excision is performed as an en-bloc excision of the skin and subcutaneous tissues over the fascial plane. It is utilized in very deep full thickness burns that are normally life threatening in nature. Important functional and cosmetic sequelae must be expected after this kind of treatment.

6.42 Fascial excision in progress. Excision is made easier by providing counter-traction.

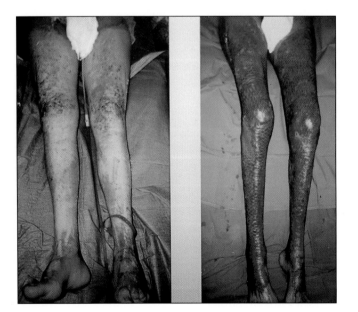

6.43 Severe contour defects result after fascial excision.

Techniques available for hemostasis
• Topical thrombin
• Topical epinephrine (adrenaline)
• Subcutaneous infiltration of epinephrine
• Fibrin glue
• Electrocautery
• Tourniquets

6.44 Different techniques are available for hemostasis. None of them has been proved to be universally effective. The technique for hemostasis has to be chosen on the basis of individual characteristics.

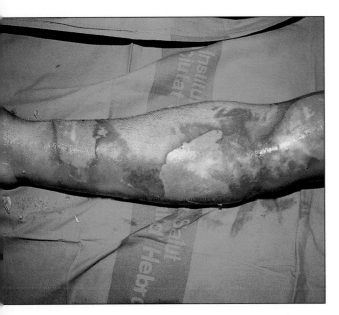

6.45 Partial thickness burns of indeterminate depth 20 days after the injury. Topical treatment was carried out initially. Burns are operated on when it is clear that they will not heal within 3 weeks.

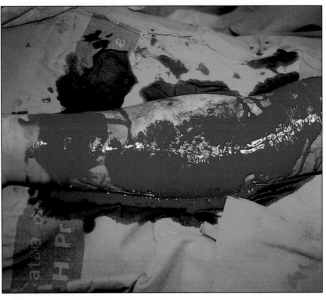

6.46 Extensive bleeding after tangential excision to living tissue in the same wound as shown in Figure 6.45.

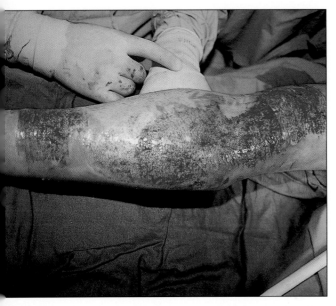

6.47 The same wound as shown in Figure 6.45 after the application of topical epinephrine (adrenaline) at a concentration of 1:10,000. Generally, complications are not usually related to topical epinephrine use during burn surgery.

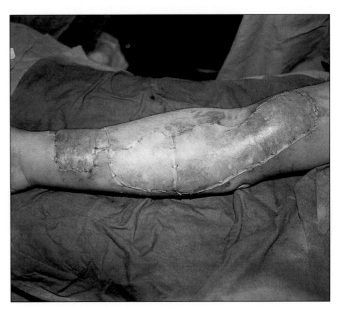

6.48 The wound is then autografted with medium thickness sheet grafts (same wound as shown in Figure 6.45).

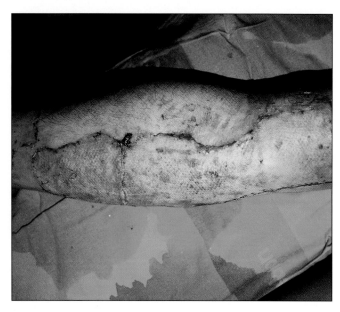

6.49 Excellent graft take 1 week after autograft in same wound as shown in Figure 6.45. With this technique, blood clots seldom occur. Extreme care must be taken to aspirate air bubbles under the graft.

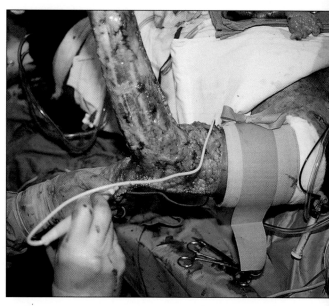

6.50 Tourniquets can be used to control blood loss during burn surgery. They can be used in either tangential or fascial excision.

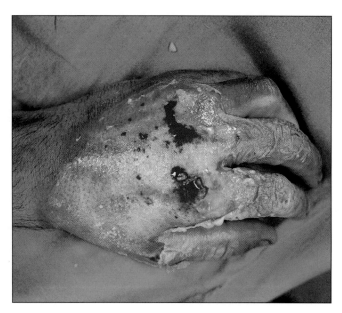

6.51 Deep second-degree contact burn to the dorsum of the hand.

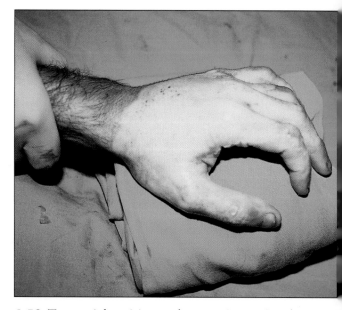

6.52 Tangential excision under tourniquet. Good experience is needed to assess viability of tissues under tourniquet, because punctate bleeding is not present.

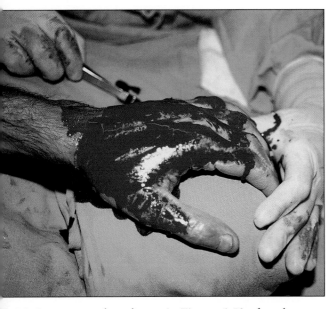

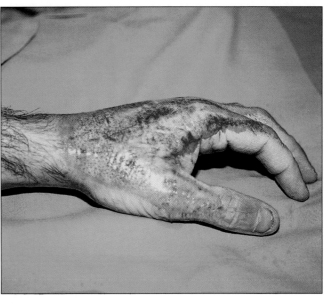

6.53 Same wound as shown in Figure 6.52 after the tourniquet has been released. Note the extensive bleeding to the area of tangential excision. It is not necessary to deflate the tourniquet if the surgeon has extensive experience with the use of tourniquets. Topical epinephrine (adrenaline) can then be applied, the area wrapped, and the tourniquet deflated.

6.54 Appearance after the application of topical epinephrine (adrenaline) 1:10,000, in the same wound as shown in Figure 6.52. Note the cadaveric appearance of the wound. Viability of tissues needs to be assessed before the topical epinephrine is applied. Afterwards, the wound takes on a cadaveric or cyanotic appearance that no longer permits viability assessment. Graft take, however, is normally excellent.

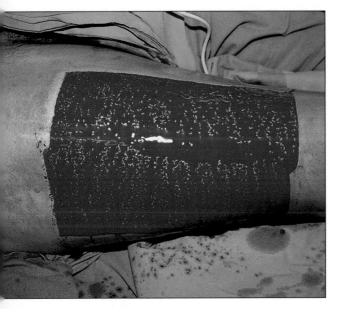

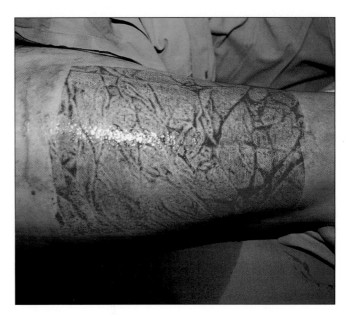

6.55 Donor sites tend to bleed extensively after skin harvesting.

6.56 Topical epinephrine (adrenaline) 1:10,000 can be applied to control donor site bleeding also, with few complications arising.

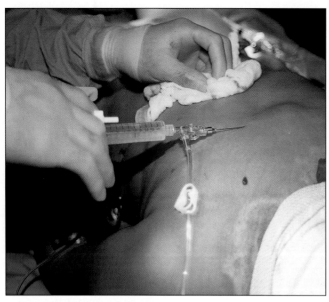

6.57 Infiltration of donor sites in the subgaleal plane in the scalp, or subcutaneous tissues in other areas (also known as 'Pitkin' technique), is very useful in smooth areas with bony prominences. It gives tension to the area, making it easier to harvest skin grafts. Epinephrine (adrenaline) at a concentration of 1:200,000 to 1:300,000 can be added to the infiltrate to control blood loss. It can also be used in areas to be excised.

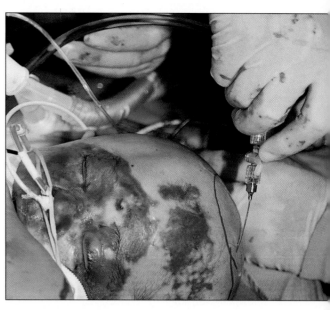

6.58 It is important to mark the hairline before shaving the scalp in order to avoid harvesting skin grafts from areas not concealed by the hair.

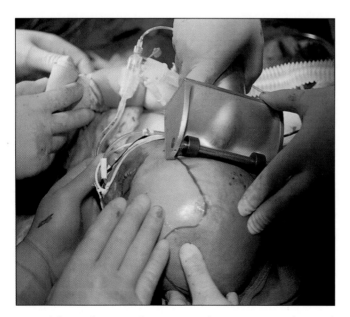

6.59 The Padgett or the Zimmer dermatome can be used for skin harvesting. Assistants should hold the donor site so tension is applied to the surrounding tissues.

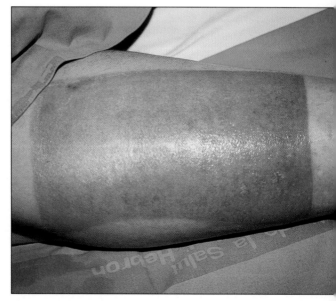

6.60 Typical appearance of a donor site 7 days after skin harvest. The hyperemic appearance disappears during the following months, but some degree of hypo-or hyperpigmentation or even scar hypertrophy may result, depending on the depth of the graft.

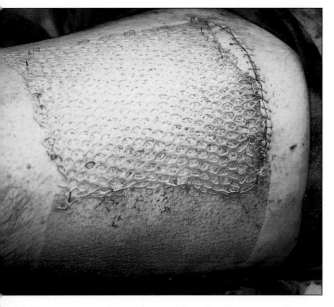

6.61 Deep donor sites taken with a depth greater than 20/1000 (0.02) of an inch can be autografted in order to decrease the healing time and prevent hypertrophic scarring.

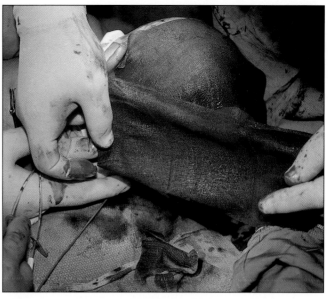

6.62 Fine-mesh gauze impregnated with scarlet red is an inexpensive treatment for the treatment of donor sites. Other treatments that can be effectively used are silver sulfadiazine, OpSite and Biobrane, depending on the size of the wound and the circumstances surrounding their acquisition.

WOUND CLOSURE

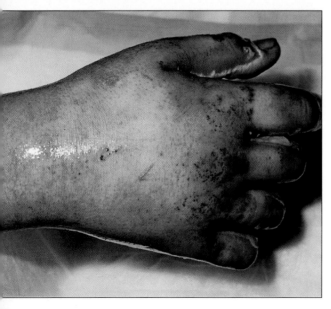

6.63 Deep second-degree burn to the dorsum of the hand and forearm caused by flame exposure.

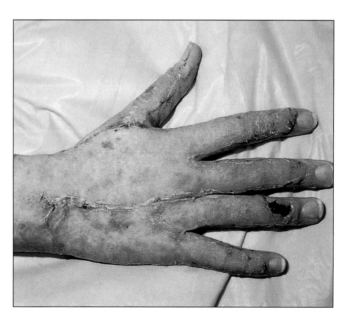

6.64 Same patient as shown in Figure 6.63 after excision and sheet autografting. Note that the seams of the grafts have been placed following the axis of the limb, so that there is no linear scarring over the knuckles.

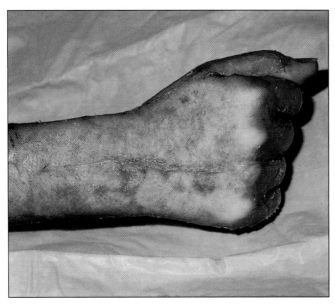

6.65 In the same patient as shown in Figure 6.63, excellent range of motion was achieved with sheet grafts and early intervention by rehabilitation services.

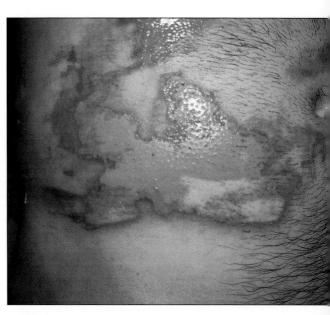

6.66 Partial thickness wounds treated conservatively for 19 days. Note that areas of deep second-degree burn have not healed.

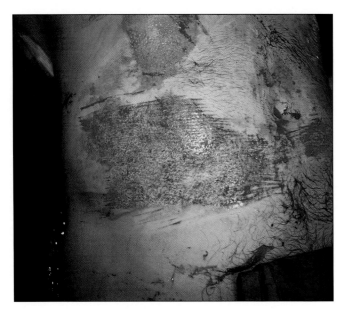

6.67 Same patient as shown in Figure 6.66 with the wounds tangentially excised and after the application of topical epinephrine (adrenaline) 1:10,000.

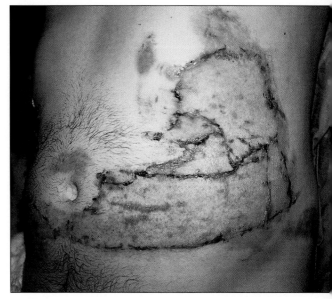

6.68 Seven days after the application of sheet grafts to the wounds in the same patient as shown in Figure 6.66. Sheet grafts should be considered first-choice treatment for burns that do not heal within 3 weeks. They provide the best cosmetic and functional outcome.

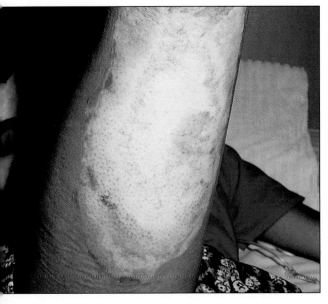

6.69 Deep second-degree burns to the popliteal fossa and posterior lower leg.

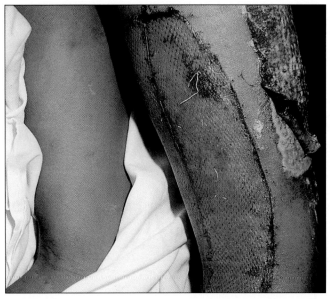

6.70 Same wound as shown in Figure 6.69 after excision and autografting with split thickness skin autografts meshed 1:1. Appearance 1 week after surgery.

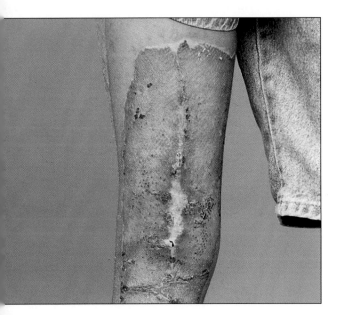

6.71 One month after the injury shown in Figure 6.69. Although meshes provide a good appearance and the slits of the 1:1 mesh prevent fluid collection, the mesh pattern stays as a permanent scar.

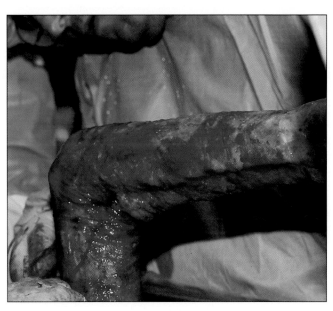

6.72 Full thickness burns to the lower extremity after excision.

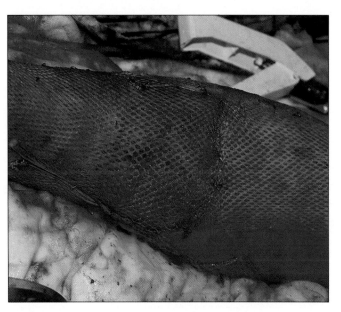

6.73 Same patient as shown in Figure 6.72 after autografting with 2:1 split thickness grafting.

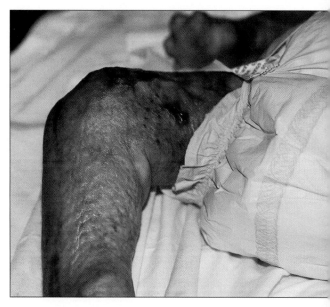

6.74 Same injury as shown in Figure 6.72, 1 month after surgery. Burn scars and mesh pattern are more noticeable than scars from sheet grafts.

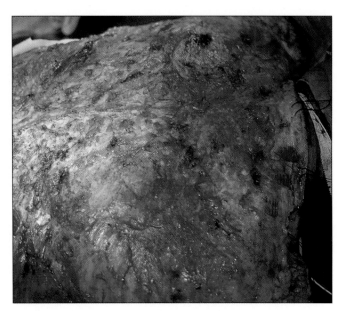

6.75 Wound to the back on a patient with a 90% total body surface area full thickness burn. Appearance after fascial excision.

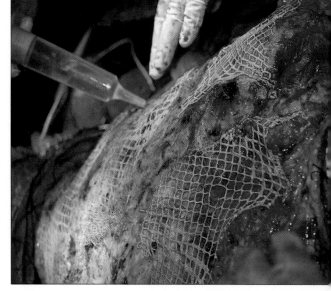

6.76 Application of 4:1 meshed autografts to the back. In mesh grafts with a mesh greater than 3:1, biologic or synthetic coverage of the interstices while the mesh pattern is closing is necessary to maintain a closed wound.

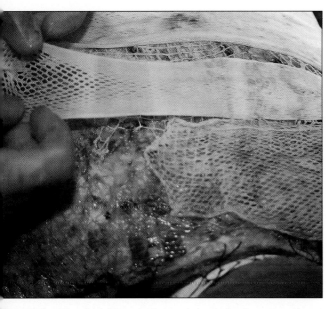

6.77 The 'Sandwich' technique. 4:1 meshed autografts are covered with 2:1 or sheet homografts as a temporary cover. Homografts desiccate when the 4:1 autograft is completely healed.

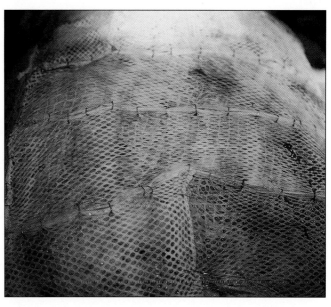

6.78 Same wound as shown in Figure 6.77 with the 'Sandwich' technique finished. The area is ready for the placement of a bolster or tied-over dressing.

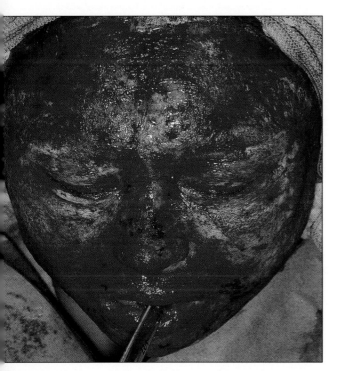

6.79 Full thickness burns to the face. Appearance after early excision.

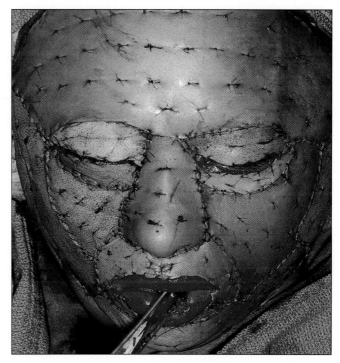

6.80 The same patient as shown in Figure 6.79 after sheet autografting to the face following esthetic units. It is very important to graft the face following these units to provide the best cosmetic outcome. Note that quilting stitches help to immobilize the grafts after surgery.

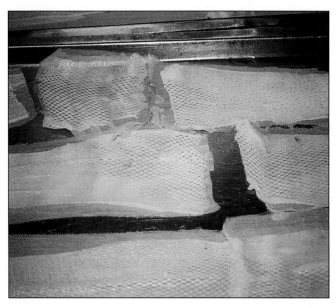

6.81 Severe burns that can not be closed with autografts after total excision, can be closed temporarily with homografts. Other options include synthetic materials and the newly available dermal substitutes.

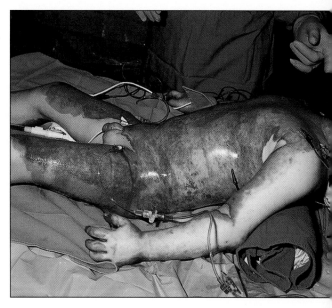

6.82 Seventy percent total body surface area flame burn in a 3-year-old patient.

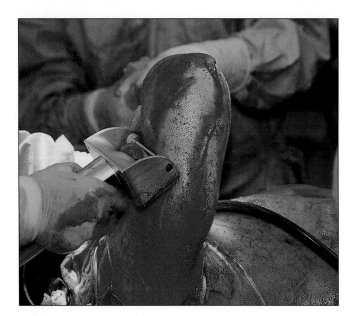

6.83 The burn wounds shown in Figure 6.82 are tangentially excised with the Padgett dermatome.

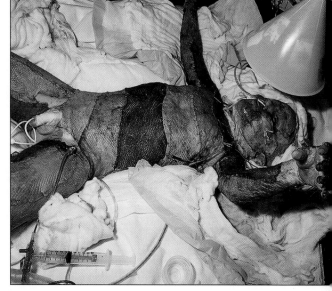

6.84 Same patient as shown in Figure 6.82 after total wound excision and closure with cryopreserved homografts. The patient was then taken to the operating theater at weekly intervals for autografting.

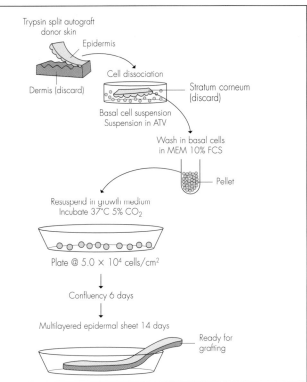

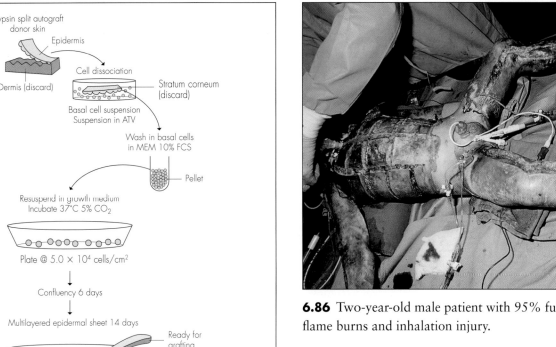

6.86 Two-year-old male patient with 95% full thickness flame burns and inhalation injury.

6.85 Basics of the culture epidermal autograft technique. In the authors' experience, the use of cultured epidermal autograft is only indicated in full thickness burns over 95% total body surface area (Adapted from Genzyme Corp).

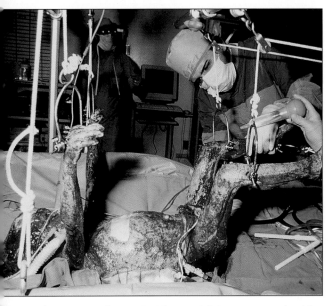

6.87 The patient shown in Figure 6.86 was treated with total wound excision within 24h of admission and homografted. Patient is shown 3 weeks after the burn. The wound is being prepared for the application of cultured keratinocytes.

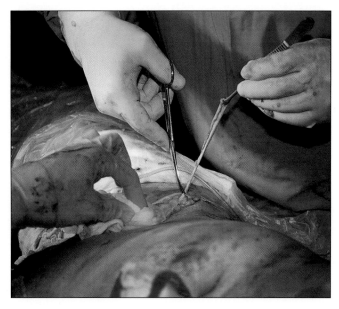

6.88 At the time of the first operative procedure, a full thickness skin biopsy is harvested and sent for culture.

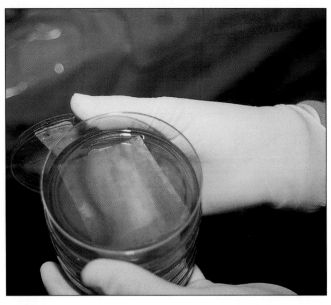

6.89 The cultured epidermal autografts are ready to use 18–21 days later. Extreme care with handling is needed because of the fragility of the cultured cells.

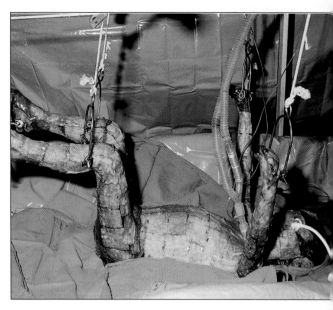

6.90 By means of cultured epidermal autograft techniques, the entire body can be covered and closed in one operative setting. Skeletal traction is used to manipulate patients after the application of cultured epidermal autograft.

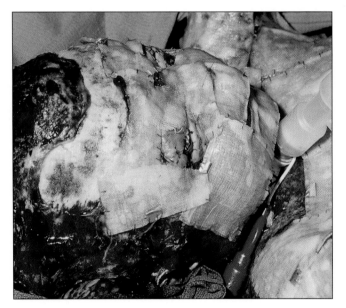

6.91 View of the face and upper extremities of the patient shown in Figure 6.86 with cultured epidermal autografts in place.

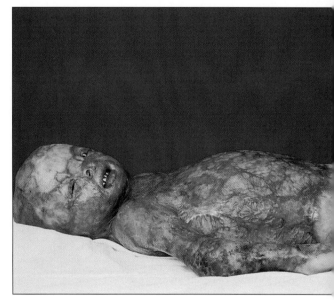

6.92 Result 5 months after the injury in the patient shown in Figure 6.86. Note the extensive sequelae of the severity of the injuries and the hypertrophic scarring and contractures typical of cultured epidermal autografts.

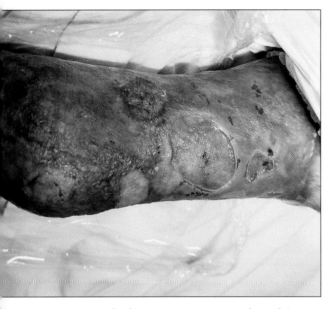

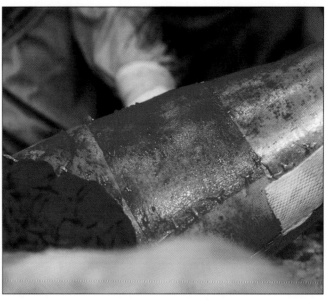

6.93 Open sore to the lower extremity in cultured epidermal autografting. Fragility of the wounds treated with cultured epidermal autografting extends for months or even years after final closure of the wounds. Extreme care is necessary to prevent blistering, but the extensive rehabilitation these patients require makes blistering and open wounds recur.

6.94 Synthetic materials, such as Trancyte, can also be used for the treatment of superficial wounds after debridement of dead tissue.

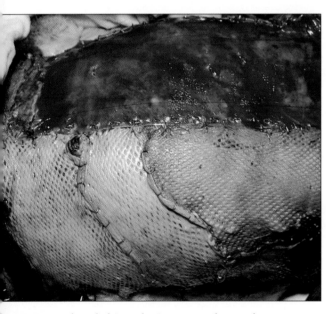

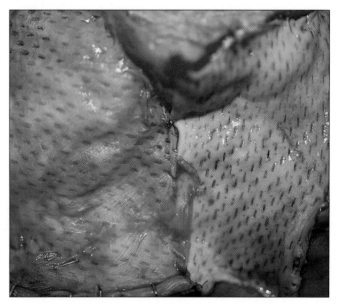

6.95 Dermal and skin substitutes can be used as temporary cover for severe burns. Integra, a bilaminar skin substitute, can replace homografts as temporary cover. The silastic superficial layer can be removed after 3 weeks and a super-thin autograft then placed on top. The entire wound can be covered with Integra, which is subsequently autografted when donor sites are available.

6.96 Other dermal substitutes are also available for wound closure. The use of AlloDerm, a commercially available human homodermis, with a super-thin autograft overlay promotes rapid healing of the donor site and re-cropping quickly becomes possible.

CHAPTER 7
INFECTIONS IN BURNS

Juan P. Barret, MD; Anthony N. Dardano, DO; and John P. Heggers, PhD

GENERAL PRINCIPLES AND MICROBIAL IDENTIFICATIONS

Burn wound infection: local signs
• Black or dark brown local areas of discoloration
• Subcutaneous tissue with hemorrhagic discoloration
• Purplish discoloration of edema of skin around the margins of the wound
• Presence of ecthyma gangrenosum
• Variable-sized abscess formation and focal subeschar inconsistency
• Partial thickness injury converted to full thickness necrosis
• Enhanced sloughing of burned tissue or eschar
• Pyocyanic appearance of subeschar tissue

7.1 The entire burn wound has to be inspected at regular intervals in order to detect any local signs of wound infection.

Microbial identification	
Methods of collection	Swabs
	Biopsies
Methods of identification	Gram stain
	Culture
	Quantitative culture
	Histopathology

7.2 Different methods are available for microbial identification and diagnosis. Swab specimens provide information regarding wound colonization. Gram stain provides an initial idea of the possible pathogen involved. When quantitative cultures with more than 10^5 colonies per gram of tissue are detected burn wound sepsis is suspected. This needs to be supported, however, by histopathologic confirmation.

Colonization and infection	
Colonization	Contamination of an open wound from the environment or from the patient himself/herself indicates microorganisms in the necrotic tissue
	This situation is dangerous, although it does not indicate an active infection
Septic burn wound	Invasion of microorganisms into viable tissue
	Localized infection without systemic spread
Burn wound sepsis	Invasion of viable tissue and systemic hematologic or lymphatic dissemination of the microorganisms themselves or their toxic products

7.3 Extreme caution has to be taken in colonized wounds, because any small alteration in the microenvironment or alterations in the host may lead to invasion and ultimately sepsis.

Clinical diagnosis of sepsis
Documentation of a septic source
And five or more of the following:
• Tachypnea (>40 breaths/min in adults)
• Prolonged paralytic ileus
• Hyperthermia (>38.5°C) or hypothermia (<36.5°C)
• Altered mental status
• Thrombocytopenia (<50,000 platelets/mm^3)
• Leukocytosis (>15.0 cells/mm^3) or leukopenia (<3.5 cells/mm^3)
• Unexplained acidosis
• Hyperglycemia

7.4 The clinical diagnosis of sepsis must be made by the documentation of a septic source, and at least five of the parameters listed.

Documentation of septic sources

- Burn wound biopsy with >10^5 organism/g tissue and/or histologic evidence of viable tissue invasion
- Positive blood culture
- Urinary tract infection with >10^5 organism/ml urine
- Pulmonary infection with positive bacteria and white cells on a class III, or better, sputum specimen

7.5 Principal sources of sepsis in burned patients. It should be noted that burn patients may acquire, at any time, any of the infections and diseases that occur in the normal population.

Principal signs of Gram-negative burn wound sepsis

Any five or more of the following provide a definitive diagnosis

- Burn wound biopsy with >10^5 organism/g tissue and/or histologic evidence of viable tissue invasion
- Rapid onset (8–12h)
- Increased temperature to 38–39°C or within normal limits (37°C)
- White blood count may be increased
- Followed by hypothermia (34–35°C) and leukopenia
- Ileus
- Hypotension and decreased urine output
- Wound develops focal gangrene
- Satellite lesions away from burn wound
- Mental obtundation

7.6 Cardinal signs in patients with gram-negative burn wound sepsis. Five or more of the listed items provide definitive diagnosis.

Principal signs of Gram-positive burn wound sepsis

Any five or more of the following provide a definitive diagnosis

- Burn wound biopsy with >10^5 organism/g tissue and/or histologic evidence of viable tissue invasion
- Symptoms develop gradually
- Increased temperature to >40°C
- White blood count increased to 20,000–50,000
- Decreased hematocrit
- Wound macerated in appearance, soupy and tenacious exudate
- Anorexic and irrational
- Ileus
- Hypotension and decreased urine output

7.7 Cardinal signs in patients with gram-positive burn wound sepsis. Five or more of the listed items provide definitive diagnosis.

BURN WOUND INFECTIONS

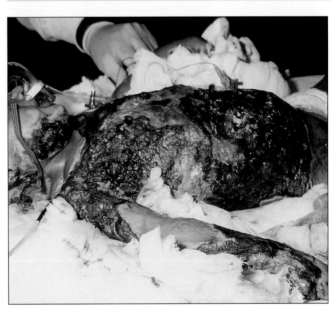

7.8 Burn wound sepsis caused by *Pseudomonas aeruginosa*. Note the dark appearance of the burn eschar. Immediate excision after resuscitation and double antibiotic coverage against all organisms identified are mandatory.

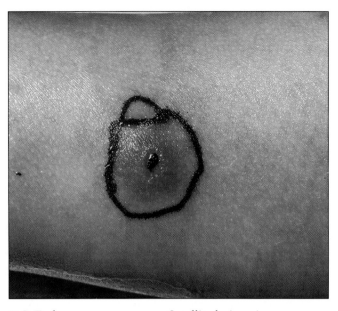

7.9 Ecthyma gangrenosum. Satellite lesions in gram-negative sepsis is typical and diagnostic.

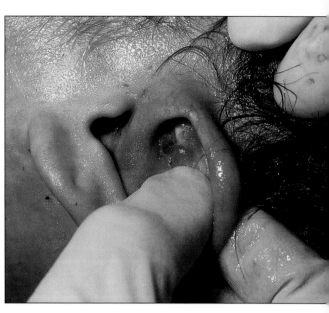

7.10 Satellite lesion to the left ear.

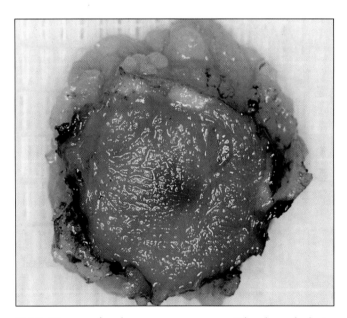

7.11 Biopsy of ecthyma gangrenosum. The thrombolytic lesion in the center of biopsy is characteristic of *Pseudomonas aeruginosa*.

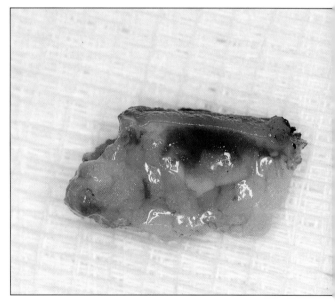

7.12 Transitional cut of biopsy showing thrombotic lesion.

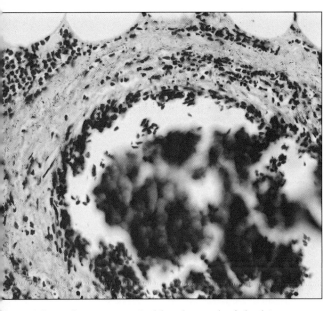

7.13 Thrombus present in blood vessel of the biopsy with bacilli in endothelium (hematoxylin and eosin, ×400).

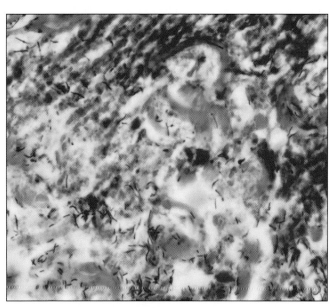

7.14 Bacilli invading deep viable tissue. Invasion of viable tissue with histopathology confirmation is currently the only way to diagnose burn wound infection (hematoxylin and eosin, ×1000).

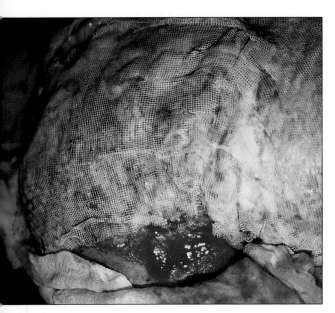

7.15 Pyocyanic discoloration on a grafted site treated with nitrofurazone ointment.

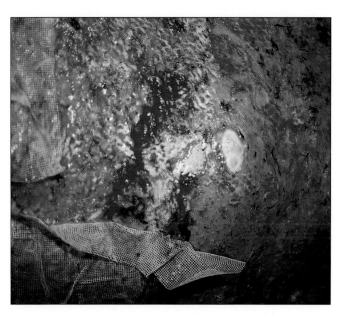

7.16 Same patient as shown in Figure 7.15 after removal of the dressings. Cultures grew *Pseudomonas aeruginosa*. Note that all autografts have disappeared as a result of the action of the bacterial enzymes.

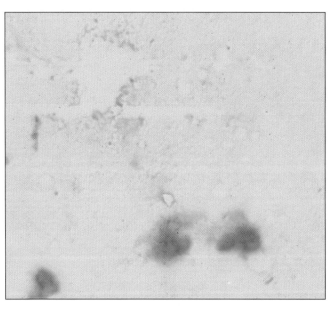

7.17 Gram stain of biopsy revealing gram-negative rods. Quantitative count 7.5×10^5 organisms per gram of tissue ($\times 1000$).

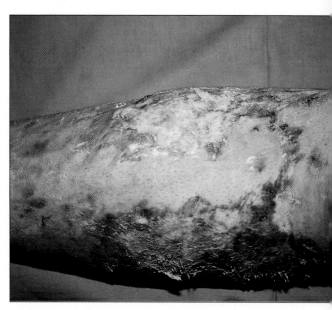

7.18 Burn wound sepsis caused by *Enterococcus* spp. The burn was initially treated with cerium nitrate silver sulfadiazine. Note the discoloration and separation of the wound.

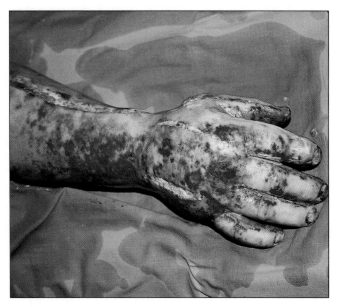

7.19 Invasive infection with *Staphylococcus* spp. The wound surface is separating and there are multiple hemorrhagic foci.

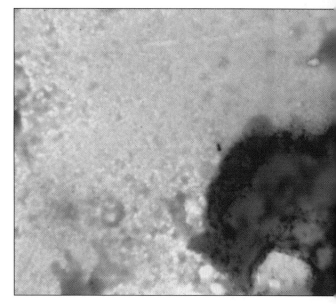

7.20 Gram stain of biopsy revealing gram-positive cocci. Quantitative count 6.2×10^5 organisms per gram of tissue ($\times 1000$).

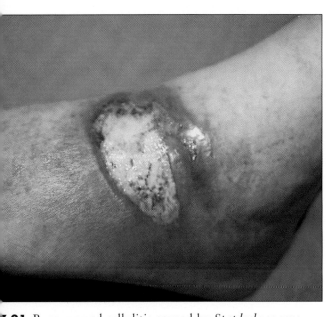

7.21 Burn wound cellulitis caused by *Staphylococcus aureus*. Clinical findings include increased pain, local inflammatory signs, and fever. Treatment includes systemic intravenous antibiotics, excision, and autografting.

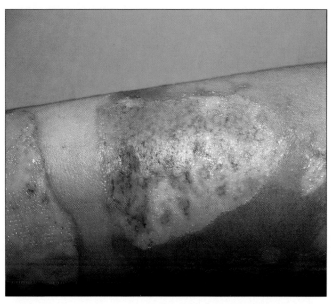

7.22 Invasive burn wound infection with *Staphylococcus aureus*. The patient presented with extreme pain, intense inflammation to the forearm, functional impairment of forearm musculature, and high fever. Immediate excision showed purulent secretions collected in the reticular dermis and subcutaneous fat.

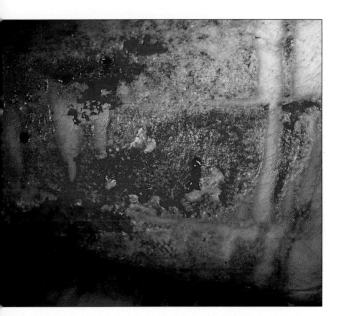

7.23 *Staphylococcus aureus* infection in donor sites. Note the secretions and the geographic appearance of the wound, which is typical of this pathogen.

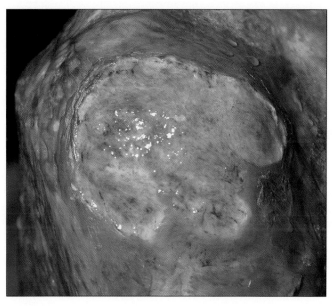

7.24 Infection of a graft site with *Staphylococcus aureus*. Prompt topical treatment with antistaphylococcal ointments or solutions stops the progression of the destruction of skin autografts.

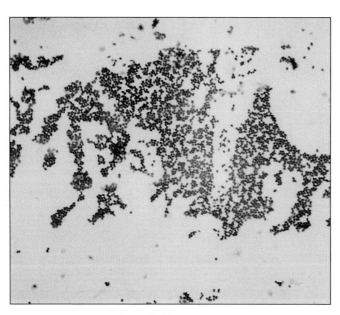

7.25 Gram stain of *Staphylococcus aureus* (×1000).

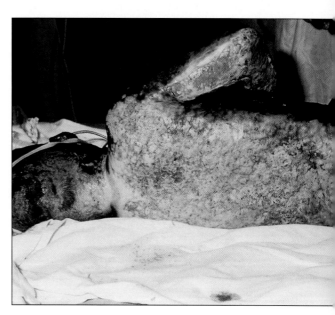

7.26 Seventy-five percent total body surface area full thickness burns with burn wound sepsis by *Enterococcus faecalis* and *Enterobacter cloacae*. Prompt excision and homografting, hemodynamic support, and systemic antibiotics controlled the infection.

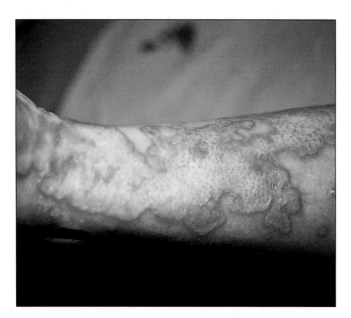

7.27 Herpes simplex virus type I infection in a patient with 35% partial thickness and full thickness burns. Extreme pain and itching are typical of this infection.

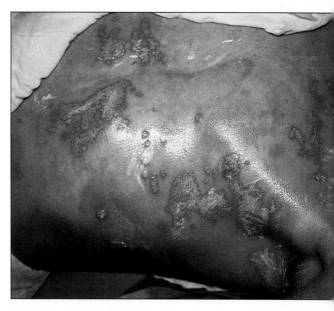

7.28 *Candida* infection in a healing second-degree burn wound. Pain and itch is usually present in this kind of infection. Treatment with silver sulfadiazine mixed with Mycostatin has proved effective in controlling *Candida* infections in burn centers.

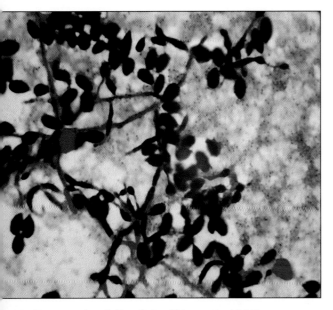

.29 Gram stain of *Candida albicans* (×1000).

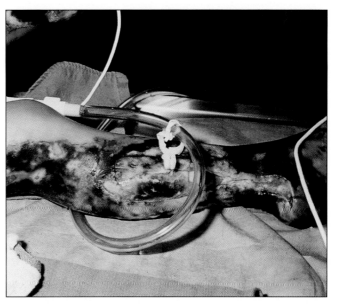

7.30 Burn wound sepsis caused by *Aspergillus* spp. Fungal infections should be suspected in wounds presenting with dark or black discoloration and hemorrhagic areas, in patients receiving prolonged systemic broad-spectrum antibiotics and/or who come from endemic areas. This patient died of fungal sepsis, fungal pneumonia, and respiratory distress syndrome.

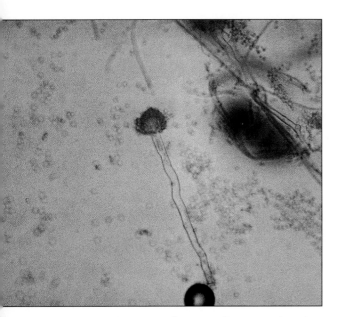

7.31 Lactophenol blue stain of *Aspergillus* sp. isolated from a burn wound biopsy (×400).

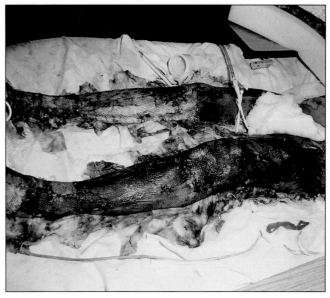

7.32 Fungal burn wound sepsis. Systemic antifungals, topical nystatin powder, and excision of all affected areas, which usually includes fascial excision and amputations, is the treatment of choice for such deadly infections.

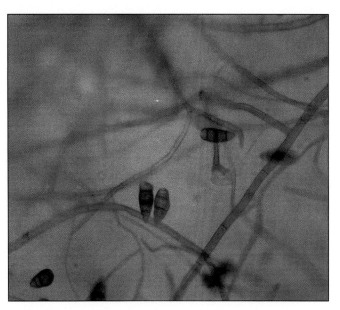

7.33 Lactophenol blue stain of a fungus from a burn wound biopsy identified as *Curvularia* spp. (×400).

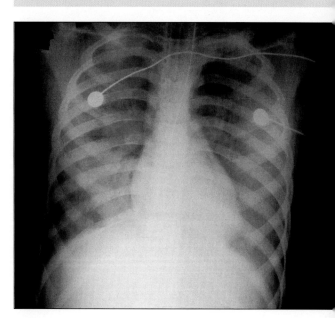

7.34 This radiograph shows massive alveolar pneumonia. Although death by sepsis is declining in burn patients, respiratory infections are still a great concern, especially in patients with inhalation injury.

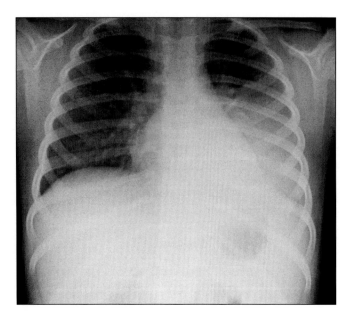

7.35 Left lower pneumonia. Burn patient with typical radiographic picture of lobar pneumonia. The diagnosis of pneumonia in patients with inhalation injury and respiratory distress syndrome is still very difficult.

Diagnosis of pneumonia in the burn intensive care unit

- Fever (or substantial change in the fever pattern of the patient)
- Leukocytosis (or substantial change in the acute hematologic response of the patient)
- Productive cough (if not intubated)
- Substantial change in the quantity and purulence of sputum
- Need for an increase in the amount of ventilatory support
- A new or changed pattern of infiltrates on chest radiography
- Decline in the patient's clinical condition without another identifiable source
- Class III sputum or better with organisms and more than 20 white blood cells per low power field

7.36 Criteria for the diagnosis of pneumonia in the burn intensive care unit setting.

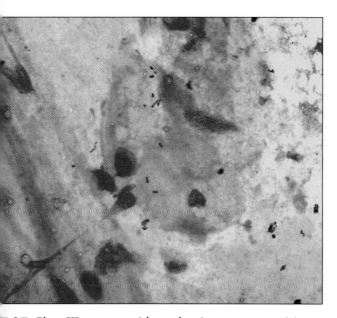

7.37 Class III sputum with predominant gram-positive organisms. The number of epithelial cells and neutrophils should be quantified under low power (×100) in order to maximize the diagnostic yield. Samples with more than 25 neutrophils and fewer than 10 epithelial cells contain minimal oropharyngeal contamination (Gram stain ×1000).

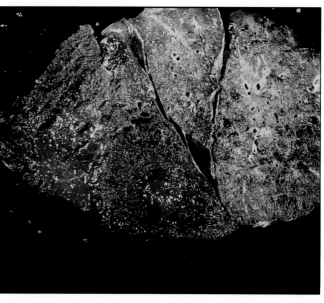

7.38 Lower lobe pneumonia superimposed on a severe respiratory distress syndrome.

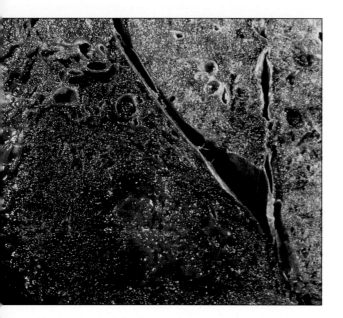

7.39 Closer view of the lesion shown in Figure 7.38, which presents with a central area of hemorrhagic necrosis.

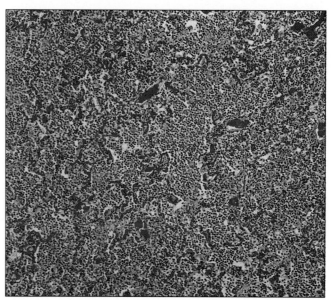

7.40 Microscopic examination of the same area as shown in Figure 7.38 showing an intense inflammatory infiltrate to the lung parenchyma (hematoxylin and eosin, ×100).

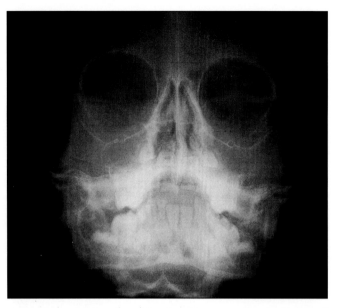

7.41 Suppurative sinusitis after long-term intubation and tracheostomy. Note that the pneumatization of maxillary sinuses has disappeared bilaterally.

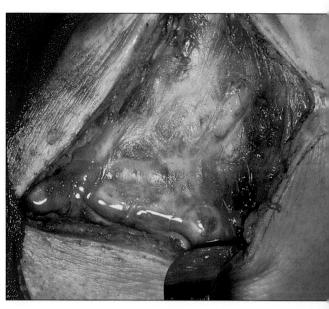

7.42 Close-up view of infected intravenous site at ankle with suppurative thrombophlebitis. This patient with lower extremity IV access developed fever, leukocytosis, and erythema at the intravenous site.

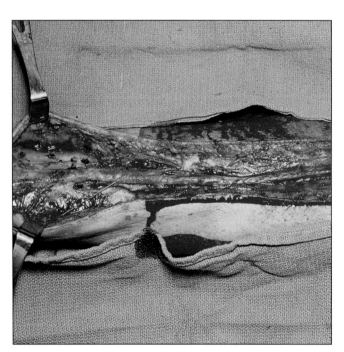

7.43 In the same patient as shown in Figure 7.42, suppurative infection was noted along the length of vein. Proper treatment is total excision of vein from the site of infection to the point of entry into central circulation.

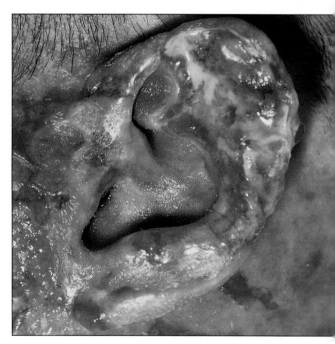

7.44 Left ear with suppurative chondritis. Chondritis seen 3 weeks after flame burn to left ear. Note the erythema and drainage from the helical rim.

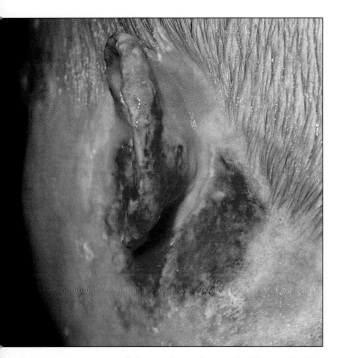

7.45 Posterior view of the patient shown in Figure 7.44. Patients usually complain of dull pain, with warmth and tenderness to the touch. Topical mafenide acetate is the treatment of choice.

Common sites of infection in burn patients
• Burn wound infection
• Pneumonia
• Cannula infections and suppurative thrombophlebitis
• Suppurative chondritis
• Suppurative sinusitis
• Urinary tract infections
• Subacute bacterial endocarditis

• Intra-abdominal infections
    Regional enteritis
    Necrotizing enterocolitis
    Acute cholecystitis
    Cholangitis

7.46 Usual sites to be investigated in burn patients who develop sepsis.

Common pathogens involved in infections in burn patients	
Gram-positive bacteria	Streptococcal infections Staphylococcal infections Enterococcal infections
Gram-negative bacteria	*Pseudomonas aeruginosa* *Escherichia coli* *Klebsiella pneumoniae* *Enterobacter cloacae*
Fungi	*Candida* spp. Filamentous fungi
Viruses	Cytomegalovirus Varicella-zoster infection Herpes simplex

7.47 Common pathogens involved in infections in burn patients. It should be remembered that other pathogens may be included or excluded depending on the local flora of each burn center.

CHAPTER 8
COMPLICATIONS

Juan P. Barret, MD; Anthony N. Dardano, DO; and David N. Herndon, MD

LOCAL COMPLICATIONS

Open Wounds, Grafts, And Donor Sites

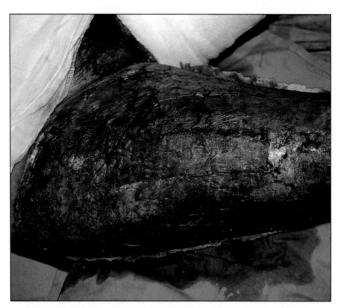

8.1 Hematomas under autografts are one of the causes of graft loss. Shearing forces, accumulation of seromas, air bubbles, and infections are other factors that can lead to graft failure. Any collection that interposes between the wound bed and the dermal side of the graft will prevent the inosculation of capillary vessels.

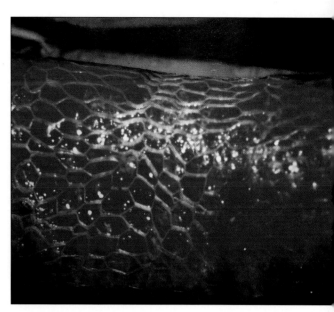

8.2 Wound with granulating tissue grafted with 3:1 meshed autografts.

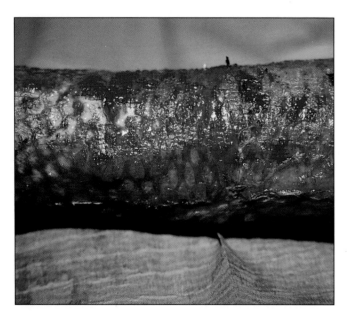

8.3 The same wound as shown in Figure 8.2, 5 days after autografting. The mesh pattern is still visible, but the autograft is melting or vanishing. The melting graft syndrome or ghosting graft syndrome is probably related to the action of collagenases that are present in chronic wounds and wounds colonized by bacteria.

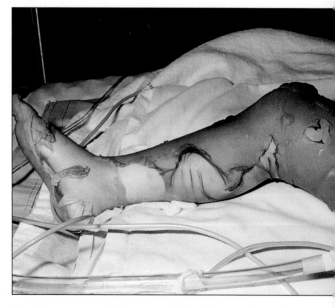

8.4 Deep second-degree and third-degree flame burns to the lower extremities. The patient was treated with immediate excision and autografting.

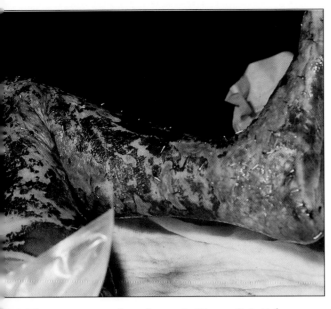

8.5 The same wound as shown in Figure 8.4, 5 days later. Some grafts are melting due to inadequate excision of small areas. Human collagenases dissolve the remaining burn eschar and part of the autografts.

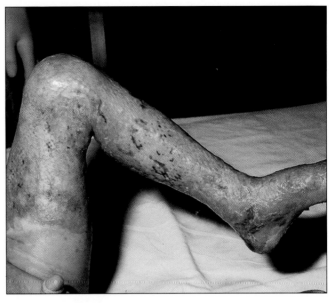

8.6 The same patient as shown in Figure 8.5, 1 week later after treatment with silver nitrate solution. The melting or ghosting syndrome can be treated with different dressings, such as silver nitrate, normal saline, Dakin's solution, and Bactroban ointment.

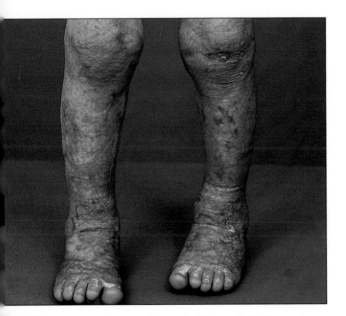

8.7 The same patient as shown in Figure 8.4, 5 months after the injury.

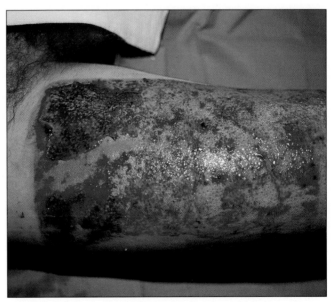

8.8 Hematoma and infection of a donor site. Excellent wound care must be applied to donor sites to avoid complications. Prolonged healing may lead to hypertrophy and pigmentation changes. In severe burns, donor site complications can lead to serious problems for definitive wound closure. In some circumstances donor sites may convert to full thickness loss.

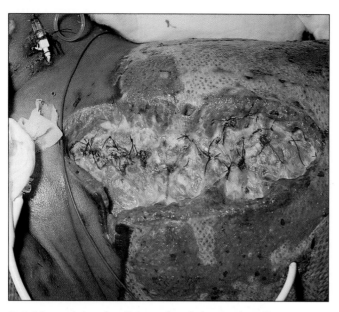

8.9 Necrotizing fasciitis to the abdominal wall.

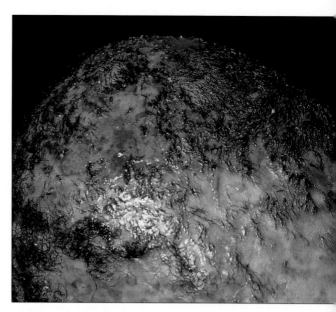

8.10 Chronic folliculitis to the scalp, also known as the concrete scalp deformity. Hairs from hair-bearing areas are embedded in the granulation tissue of converted second-degree burns and donor sites, and micro-organisms are entrapped prolonging the process. Shaving of the affected area, topical treatment and eventually skin autografting resolve the problem.

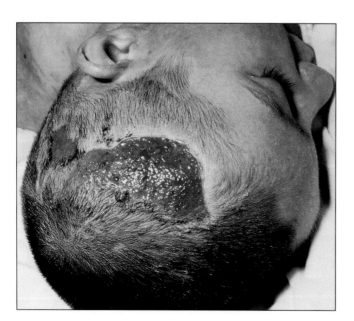

8.11 Donor site converted to full thickness loss.

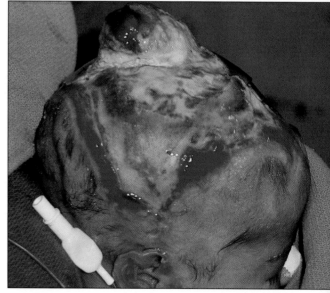

8.12 Cerebral herniation through full thickness burn to the scalp, calvaria, and meninges. Urgent closure of the wound is mandatory when this complication occurs. Cerebral abscesses are a probable late complication.

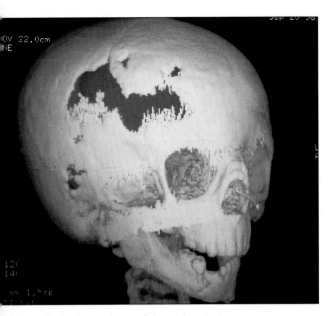

8.13 Full thickness loss of the calvaria is a common complication of deep burns to the skull in small children. The lack of dura and/or normal brain underneath is the cause of the lack of bone formation.

Healed Wounds

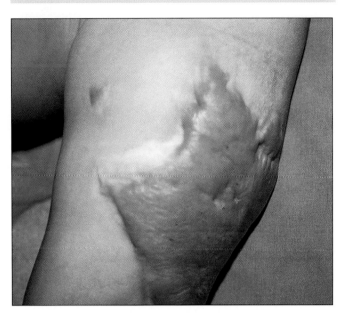

8.14 Scar hypertrophy in a healed second-degree burn. Burns, or donor sites, that require more than 3 weeks to heal are likely to develop burn scar hypertrophy. Nevertheless, individual factors may play a role in the development of scar hypertrophy.

Pressure Sores

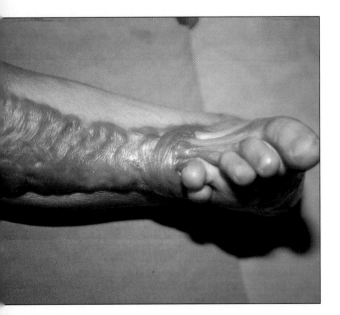

8.15 Burn scars to the lower leg and foot in a 2-year-old child. Burns were allowed to heal spontaneously. No rehabilitation was received. Neglected burns develop important contractures that prevent the affected areas from functioning normally.

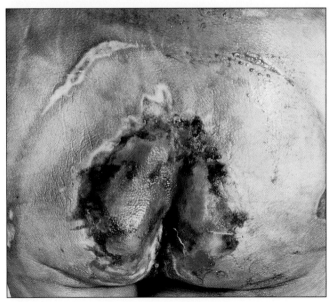

8.16 Sacral pressure sore in a patient with severe burns. Severely burned patients with prolonged bed rest require frequent rotation and positioning to prevent pressure sore postoperatively.

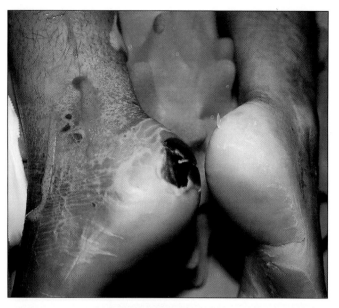

8.17 Pressure sore to the left heel. Heels and bony areas of the body need to be protected when in bed or during active physical therapy.

Pressure sore staging	
Stage I	Skin intact, but reddened
Stage II	Blister or other break in dermis
Stage III	Subcutaneous destruction to muscle
Stage IV	Involvement of bone or joint

8.18 Staging pressure sores helps to monitor healing and to plan reconstruction.

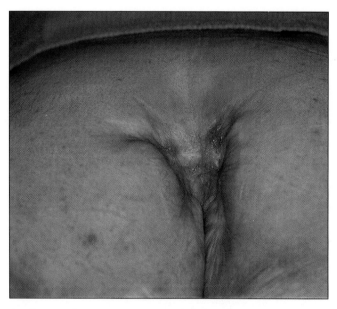

8.19 Sacral pressure sore in a burn patient. Despite air mattresses and patient rotation, pressure sores develop due to prolonged bed rest.

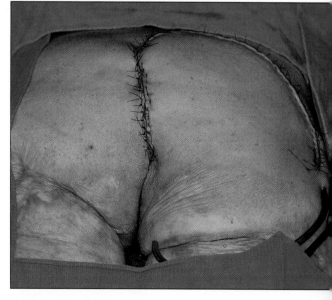

8.20 Soft tissue coverage of bony prominences is key to surgical correction of pressure sores. Here the patient had closure with a gluteal flap.

Marjolin's ulcer

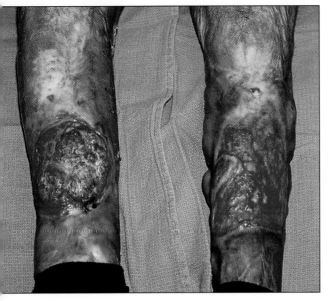

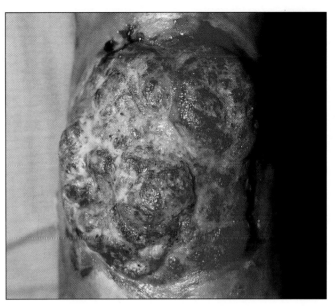

8.21 Marjolin's ulcer. This patient with 20-year-old burn wounds to the lower extremities presented with a large tumor and nonhealing wounds.

8.22 Close-up view of the tumor shown in Figure 8.21. Biopsy revealed squamous cell carcinoma.

Heterotopic Bone

8.23 Magnetic resonance imaging of the tumor shown in Figure 8.22 reveals the highly aggressive nature of this cancer.

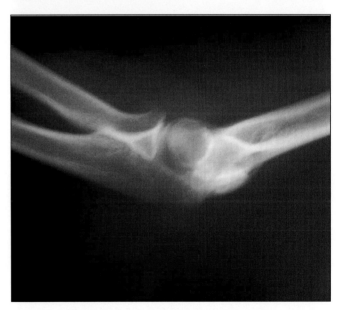

8.24 Heterotopic bone formation is a rare, but functionally important complication of thermal burns. Bed confinement and superimposed trauma to the joints are some of the determining factors for this condition. Patients who are reluctant to move joints or who have important functional limitations should be investigated for this process. Once recognized, joint exercise should be restricted to gentle passive and assisted active motion only.

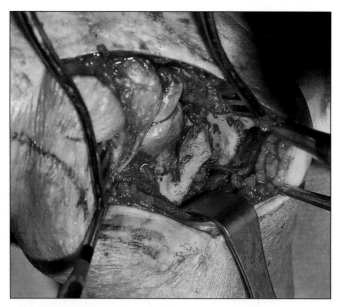

8.25 Heterotopic bone in an elbow exposed intraoperatively. Surgical excision of heterotopic bone is indicated when joint motion is lost or significantly compromised by bridging bone or exostoses.

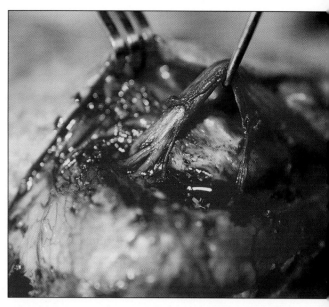

8.26 Exposure of the ulnar nerve at the level of an elbow involved in heterotopic bone formation.

GENERAL COMPLICATIONS

Cardiovascular System

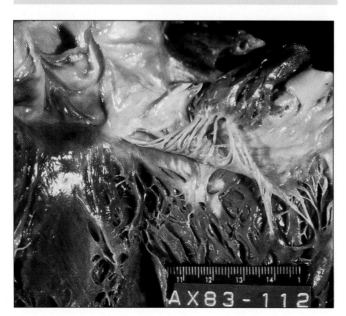

8.27 Subacute endocarditis to the tricuspid valve. Repetitive septic showers and the microtrauma of placement of central lines and Swan–Ganz catheters, put the burn patient at risk for this kind of complication.

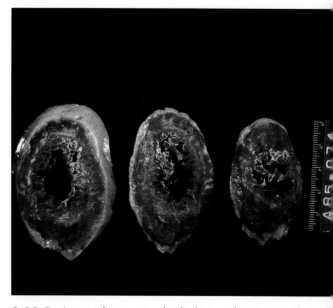

8.28 Patients who receive high doses of inotropic drug and vasopressors develop myocardial flame hemorrhages and myocardial lesions produced by chronic ischemia and hypoxia.

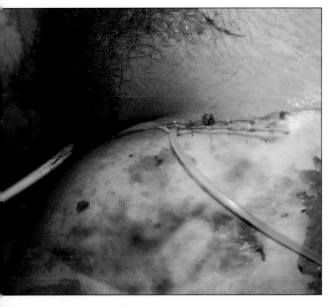

8.29 Cut-downs and femoral vein catheterization are contraindicated. They are associated with a high incidence of septic and thrombotic complications.

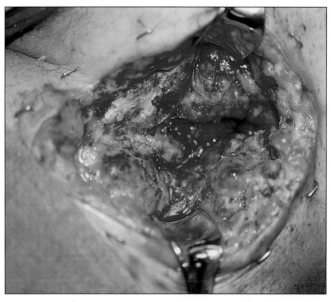

8.30 The same patient as shown in Figure 8.29, 1 week later. Intraoperative view of left femoral exploration for suppurative thrombophlebitis. The patient presented with septic thrombosis of the left common femoral vein and inferior cava vein. Ligation of the femoral vein, long-term antibiotics and anticoagulation, and placement of a Greenfield filter was necessary.

Respiratory System

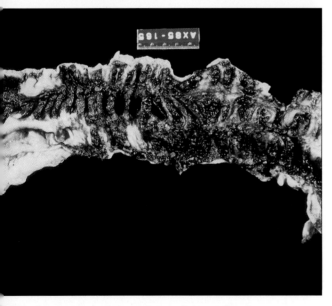

8.31 Autopsy specimen of necrohemorrhagic tracheobronchitis. Tracheobronchitis is one of the complications of inhalation injury. It can be present with or without respiratory distress. Cardinal signs are fever, leukocytosis, hoarseness, retrosternal pain, and productive cough.

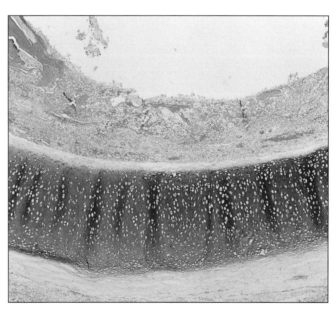

8.32 Microscopic view of specimen of tracheobronchitis. Note the destruction of the epithelium and the inflammation to the chorion. Mucous plug formation and cast formation are typical of inhalation injury. Ciliary function is also impaired, and so descendent colonization of the tracheobronchial tree is universal.

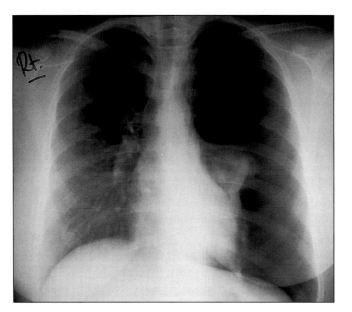

8.33 X-ray radiograph showing complete left pneumothorax secondary to barotrauma following explosion. Identification and prompt treatment is necessary. During the primary and secondary assessments, associated trauma and conditions are detected and treated.

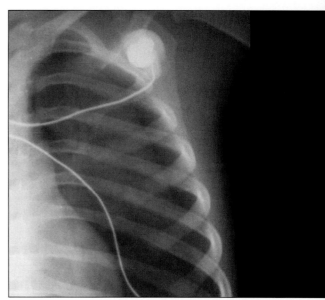

8.34 X-ray radiograph showing left pneumothorax resulting from an attempt to place a left subclavian central line. Proper treatment is tube thoracostomy in a symptomatic patient.

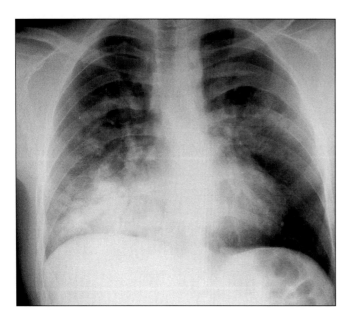

8.35 X-ray radiograph showing aspiration pneumonia in superior segment of right lower lobe. Patients who are found unconscious at the site of the accident burn incident may have aspirated.

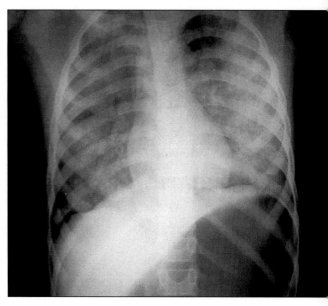

8.36 X-ray radiograph showing massive aspiration secondary to gastric dilatation. It is imperative that nasogastric intubation be performed in burn patients with burns over more than 20% total body surface area.

Gastrointestinal System

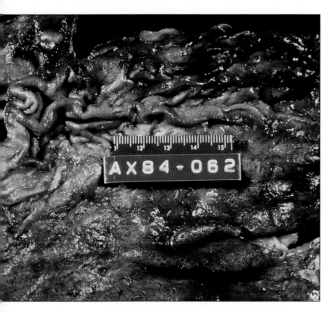

8.37 Autopsy specimen from a patient with multiple organ failure and Curling ulcer. Note the extensive ulcerations to the gastric mucosa. Prevention of gastroduodenal bleeding after thermal trauma includes prompt excision and grafting, control of the hypermetabolic response, enteral feeding by gastric and duodenal feeding, and H_2-blockers and/or sucralfate. Antacids via tube feed must be added if the pH of gastric residue is less than 5.

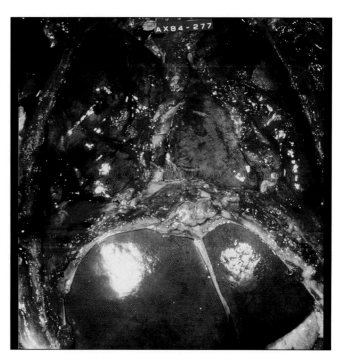

8.38 Significant enlargement of the liver and fatty deposition therein are common findings in severe and fatal burns.

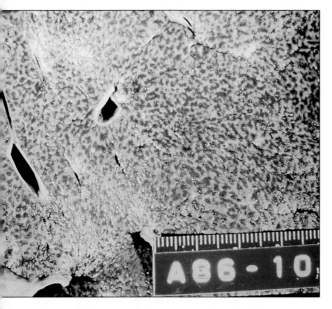

8.39 Fatty infiltration of the liver, with significant enlargement of the organ, has been related to an increased incidence of sepsis and prevention of diaphragmatic excursion with impairment of mechanical ventilation. Modulation of the hypermetabolic response and peripheral lipolysis may decrease the likelihood of occurrence of such infiltration.

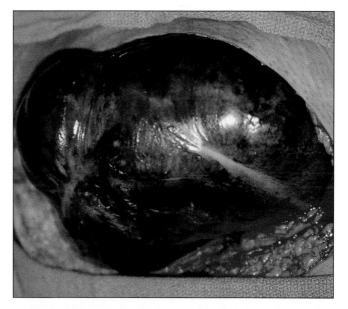

8.40 Dead sigmoid colon in an elderly burn patient with significant vascular disease. Poor visceral perfusion secondary to hypovolemia, and sepsis, can lead to bowel infarction.

Renal System

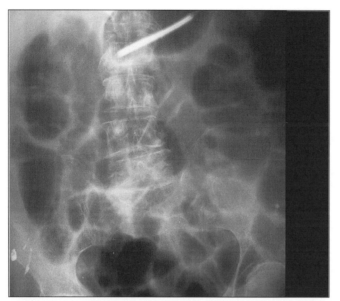

8.41 Ogilvie's syndrome in a 65-year-old female patient with a 35% total body surface area burn. Pseudo-obstruction of the colon can appear in patients receiving opioids and sedatives and in those with chronic constipation. Electrolytic imbalance has been also related to the condition. Perforation may occur and a septic appearance with profound acidosis can be present. Decompression in severe cases is mandatory. If double lumen air lines or free air is present in plain radiograph, surgical exploration and resection are necessary.

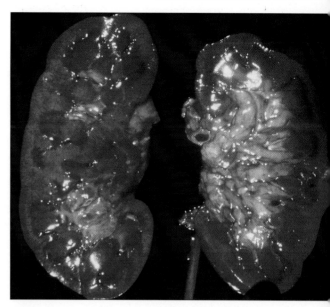

8.42 Autopsy specimens from a patient with acute tubular necrosis and renal failure. Note the edema and the alteration of medullary pyramids. Acute renal failure in burn patients carries a high mortality.

Management of renal failure in burn patients	
Hemofiltration device not required	Fluid balance (central venous pressure and/or pulmonary capillary wedge monitoring is necessary) Diuretics (not in established organic renal failure) Management of hyperkalemia (ion-exchange resins, 10% dextrose + insulin, sodium bicarbonate, calcium chloride in severe cases with serum potassium above 6.0mmol/l)
Hemofiltration device required	Peritoneal dialysis Hemoperfusion Hemodialysis

8.43 Techniques available for the management of renal failure in burn patients. Although hemodialysis is recommended by many, it is sometimes very difficult to maintain a stable circulation with this technique. In addition, the anticoagulation required for hemodialysis may be a problem in open wounds and bleeding through burns. Peritoneal dialysis is an excellent alternative in the authors' experience, especially in burn-injured children.

Criteria for hemodialysis in burn patients
• Blood urea nitrogen > 70mg/dl
• Creatinine >5mg/dl
• Potassium >6mmol/l
• Base excess <−15mmol/l
• Pulmonary edema
• Systemic signs of uremia

8.44 Criteria for the introduction of hemodialysis to treat acute renal failure in burn patients.

Multiple Organ Failure

Cascades of multiple organ failure	
Early cascade of multiple organ failure in burn patients	Resuscitation failure Respiratory distress syndrome Hemodynamic failure Renal failure Liver failure Intestinal failure Infection Vasomotor failure and death
Late cascade of multiple organ failure in burn patients	Pulmonary failure Hemodynamic instability Renal failure Intestinal failure Liver failure Vasomotor failure and death

8.45 The sequence of multiple organ failure often follows a predictable course, although the cascade can be modified by different treatments. In burn patients, two cascades have been described, an early and a late cascade. Mortality increases with increasing numbers of failed organ systems. When three organs have failed, mortality has been reported as 100%.

Etiology of multiple organ failure in burn patients
• The wound
• Sepsis
• Intestinal barrier failure
• Inadequate organ perfusion

8.46 Once established, multisystem organ failure is very difficult to reverse, emphasizing the importance of prevention. Preventive measures are based on our crude understanding of the mechanisms that drive the process.

CHAPTER 9
PREVENTION AND TREATMENT OF DEFORMITY IN BURN PATIENTS

Peter Dziewulski, FRCS, FRCS (Plast); Juan P. Barret, MD; and David N. Herndon, MD

GENERAL PRINCIPLES AND CLINICAL FEATURES

Prevention of burn deformities

- Proper positioning with or without splints
- Exercise to maintain range of motion in joints
- Maintenance of muscle strength and muscle tone
- Early mobilization

9.1 Burn trauma requires immediate aggressive intervention by rehabilitation services to prevent debilitating deformities. Burn distribution as well as burn depth are good predictors of rehabilitation outcomes.

Position of comfort/contracture in burn patients

- Neck flexion
- Shoulder protraction
- Elbow flexion
- Metacarpal extension
- Interphalangeal flexion
- Wrist flexion
- Hip flexion
- Knee flexion
- Ankle plantar flexion

9.2 The position of comfort/contracture needs to be avoided, because this is responsible for many of the deformities encountered in burn patients. Positioning in bed, splinting, and active movements help to prevent deformities.

Causes of deformities to the spine

- Unilateral or asymmetric burns to the trunk, neck, axillae, or groins can cause lateral curvature of the spine
- Burns to the anterior chest and neck can cause exaggerated kyphosis
- Severe deep burns to the abdomen can interfere with abdominal muscle function resulting in an increased lordosis

---

9.3 Deformities to the spine can be caused by intrinsic unilateral burn scars to the trunk or deformities to the adjacent joints.

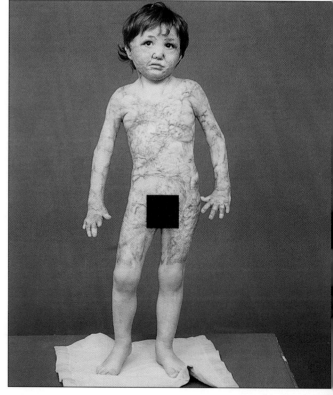

9.4 Three-year-old male patient affected by burn scars to the trunk and contracture of the right groin that is causing lateral curvature of the spine.

Functional impairments that result from burns to the neck, shoulder girdle, and axillae

• Bridging scars from chin to neck to anterior shoulders result in:
    Exaggerated kyphosis
    Neck flexion
    Protraction of the shoulders
 • Severe functional impairment of shoulder flexion and independence

9.5 Burns that cross joints and affect the shoulder and the upper extremities are more functionally debilitating.

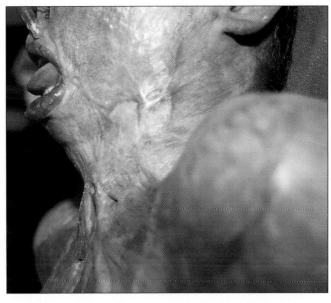

9.6 Severe burn scar contracture to the anterior neck that bridges the chin and anterior chest resulting in shoulder protraction and kyphosis. The patient required several burn scar releases in order to acquire complete normal function.

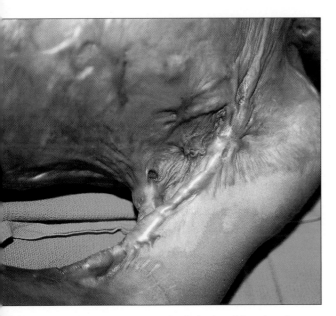

9.7 Burn scar contracture to the left shoulder that is producing a severe disability to the upper extremity.

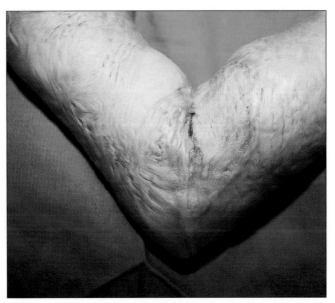

9.8 Severe burns of the upper extremity often result in keeping the elbow in the position of comfort, which is flexion.

> **Physical deformities that result from burns to the wrist and hand**
>
> - The 'burned hand position' often involves
>   Wrist flexion
>   Metacarpophalangeal extension
>   Interphalangeal flexion
>   First metacarpal extension and adduction
> - Overall appearance of the hand is that of a 'claw deformity'

9.9 Burns to the hands that do not receive proper rehabilitation, result in an extremely debilitating deformity.

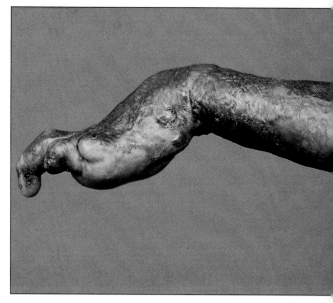

9.10 Typical claw deformity in a burn patient. Proper positioning and splinting during the acute phase and intensive exercise programs can prevent the occurrence of such deformities.

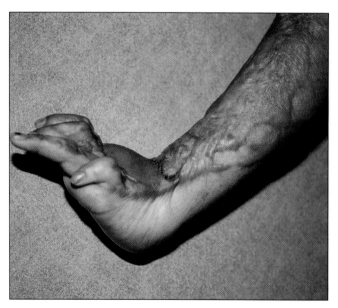

9.11 When burn scars exist only on the dorsum of the wrist, hand, and forearm, an extension deformity to the wrist results.

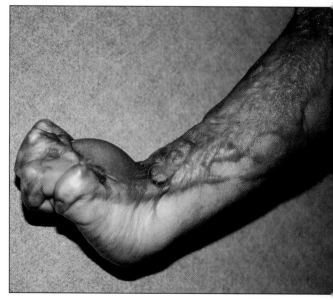

9.12 Same patient as shown in Figure 9.11 with full flexion of the fingers and wrist. Note that the disability is very significant.

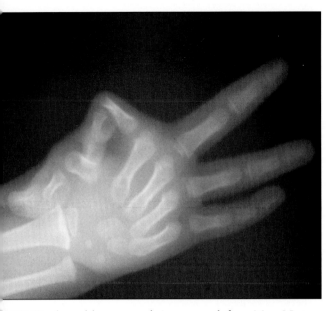

9.13 Neglected burns result in severe deformities. Note the severe deformity to the thumb and index fingers.

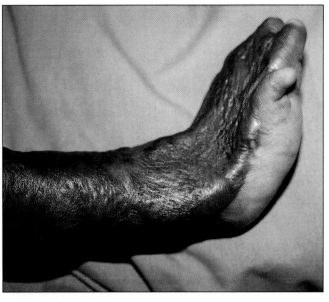

9.14 Dorsal deformity to the hand and partial amputation of all of the fingers, rendering the hand useless.

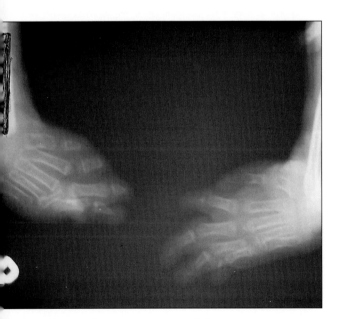

9.15 Radiographic examination of the same patient as shown in Figure 9.14.

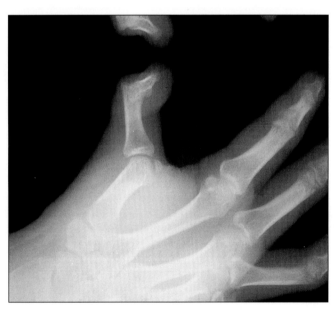

9.16 Subluxation of the first metacarpophalangeal joint secondary to severe burn scar contracture.

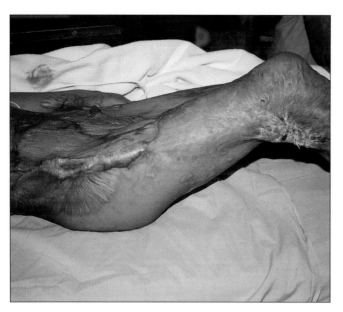

9.17 Hip flexion and knee flexion is the position of comfort for these joints. Bilateral involvement of hip joints results in increased lumbar lordosis and/or knee flexion.

Physical deformities that result from burns to the foot and ankle

- The most common deformity that occurs in deep burns is equinovarus deformity. It includes:
  Ankle equinus
  Hind-foot inversion
  Forefoot varus and equinus

- Intrinsic deformities of the foot occur from extreme extension of the toes from dorsal foot burns

- Rocker bottom foot occurs when both anterior and posterior scars are present

9.18 Principal deformities to the foot and ankle region. Proper position during recovery is essential to maintain normal gait.

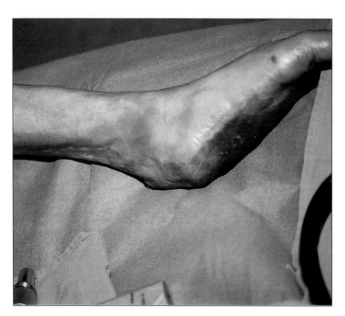

9.19 Equinovarus deformity of the left foot. Deformity results from ill-positioned joints during the recovery phase and neglected contractures.

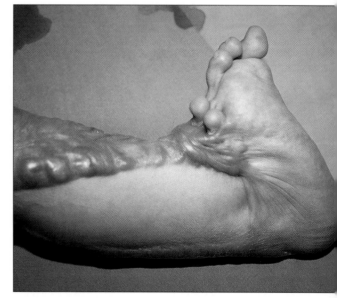

9.20 Neglected dorsal contractures to the foot result in severe deformities and functional impairment.

POSITIONING, EXERCISE, AND AMBULATION

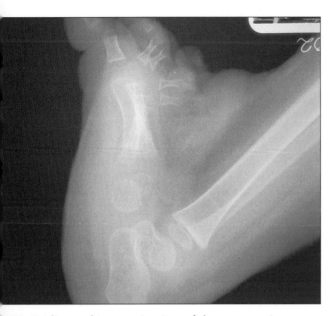

9.21 Radiographic examination of the same patient as shown in Figure 9.20. Note that all joints are hyperextended.

Appropriate positioning in bed
• Maintain straight alignment of the trunk and neck
• Neck should be in slight extension
• Arms should be elevated in the neutral plane or in line with the glenoid, with 15–20° horizontal flexion and 80° of abduction
• Elbow in full extension
• Hand in the intrinsic plus position with the thumb in flexion and abduction
• Hips in extension and abduction
• Knees in full extension
• Foot in neutral position and 90° or greater dorsiflexion

9.22 Positioning the patient in bed in the correct position is essential to avoid later reconstructive problems. The position also needs to be tailored to individual patient needs, because the specific location and severity of the injuries play an important role in the rehabilitation process.

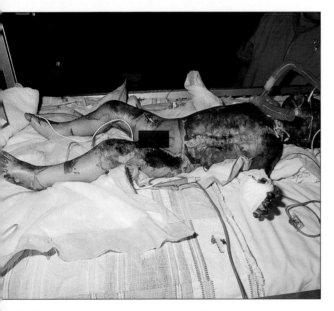

9.23 Burn trauma produces the position of comfort, which results, if not rectified, in burn deformities. Note the knee and hip flexion, and the equinovarus position of the feet in this severely burned patient.

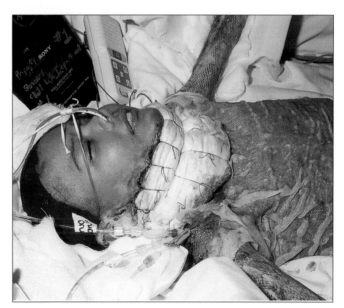

9.24 Positioning the patient in bed is essential to produce the best outcome. All joints need to be assessed and repositioned as necessary.

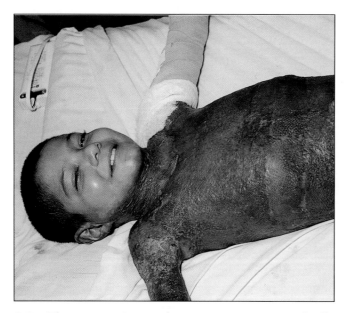

9.25 The same patient as shown in Figure 9.24, with all burns healed. Note the good result of axillary and neck burns.

Benefits of early mobilization/ambulation

- Helps to maintain range of motion
- Maintains strength in the lower extremities
- Prevents thromboemboliism
- Assists in maintaining bone density through weight bearing
- Promotes independence through recreational and functional activities

9.26 All patients, regardless of burn size, location, and severity, must be started on a program of early mobilization and ambulation.

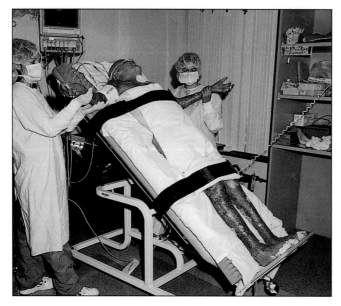

9.27 Early mobilization, ambulation, and exercise are part of acute care and rehabilitation. Protocol of early mobilization and ambulation can begin as soon as the patient is deemed stable. Wounds need to be properly dressed and lower extremities double wrapped with elastic bandages to insure capillary support.

Goals of exercise

- Reduction of edema
- Maintenance of joint motion
- Maintenance of strength
- Reduction of scar
- Maintenance of developmental level
- Maintenance of independence in activities of daily living
- Maintenance of mobiliity

9.28 A Exercise is painful and tedious. It should begin as soon as possible, with isometric exercises if the patient has received autografts, and an aggressive active program if conservative treatment for burn wounds is in effect.

Movements to counteract the position of comfort/contracture	
Neck	Extension, lateral flexion, rotation
Shoulder	Flexion, abduction
Elbow	Extension, supination
Metacarpal	Flexion
Interphalangeal	Extension
Wrist	Extension
Knee	Extension
Ankle	Dorsiflexion
Metatarsal	Flexion

9.28 B Exercise should be addressed to counteract the position of confort/contracture.

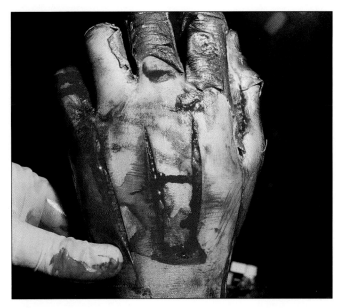

9.29 Full thickness burns to the dorsal and palmar aspects of the hand in a patient with 85% total body surface area burns.

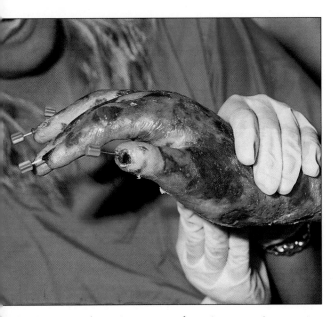

9.30 Active and passive range of motion exercises start as soon as possible to maintain range of motion in joints not internally fixed.

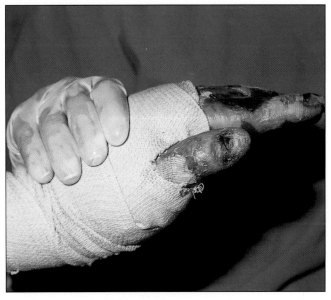

9.31 Proper positioning when at rest is also very important for the rehabilitation program.

General principles of splinting	
Splint utilization	Immobilization Mobilization
Types of splints	Static Dynamic
Wearing schedule	At all times immediately post-op Nights only as active range of motion increases

9.32 Positioning and splinting positively relieves many of the problems faced in the care of burn patients. Besides splints, other positioning devices include arm troughs, sky hooks, and slings.

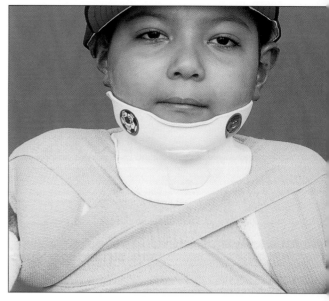

9.33 Hard neck collar in place to prevent anterior neck contractures. Note that the patient is also wearing a figure-of-eight bandage to prevent shoulder adduction and flexion.

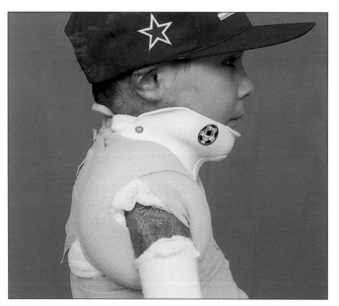

9.34 Neck collars must be worn at all times when not exercising. If there are grafted areas on the chest, they must be protected. When scars on the neck exist, patients should sleep without a pillow in order to maximize neck extension (same patient as shown in Figure 9.33).

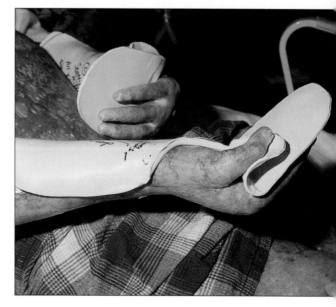

9.35 Hands have to be splinted in the intrinsic-plus position with the thumb flexed and abducted. In this position, all collateral ligaments are stretched.

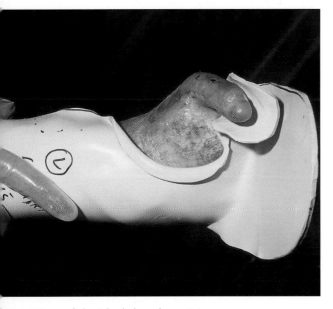

9.36 View of the ideal thumb position.

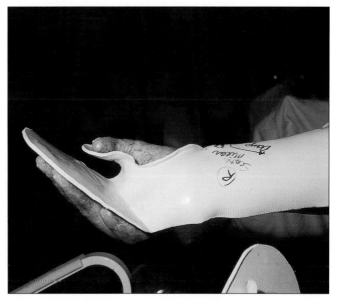

9.37 Splints can be fabricated on admission and applied immediately. Bony areas need to be protected and loose dressings should be used to hold the splints in place, but they should be tight enough to avoid exposing graft to shearing forces.

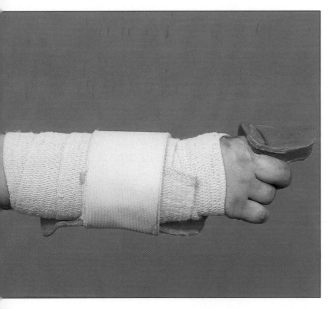

9.38 When only some parts of the limb, hand, or other anatomic area have been injured, all uninjured areas may be left nonsplinted so that active exercise can be performed with that joint.

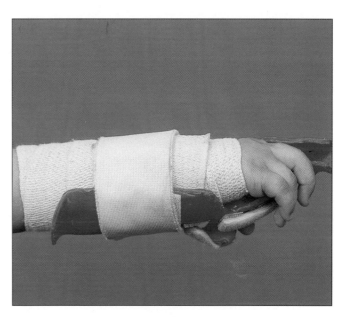

9.39 Note that the third, fourth, and fifth fingers can be exercised, maintaining the thumb and index fingers splinted (same patient as shown in Figure 9.38).

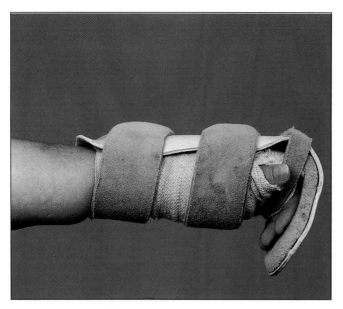

9.40 When a specific deformity exists, custom-made splints for each specific patient must be fabricated to counteract the forces of the deformity. Note how the splint is fabricated to oppose the forces of a dorsal contracture to the metacarpophalangeal joints.

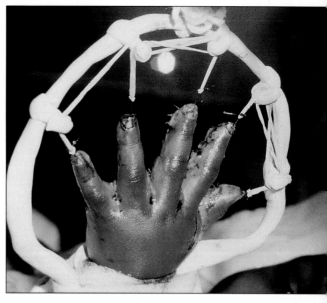

9.41 The ukulele splint is useful to manage exposed grafts to the hand and maintain active range of motion in the fingers. Note that fingers are fixed with rubber bands, so that only active movements can mobilize the hand.

SKELETAL FIXATION AND TRACTION

9.42 Mouth spreaders are also very helpful to maintain the width of the mouth in patients at risk for microstomia. The splint must be worn at all times except when eating.

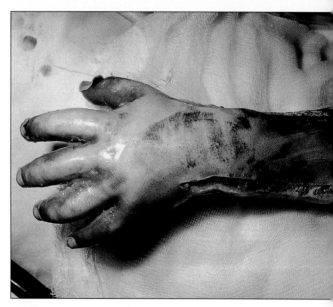

9.43 Severe burns involving deep structures and joint and/or tendon structures, benefit from temporary internal fixation with K-wires for positioning.

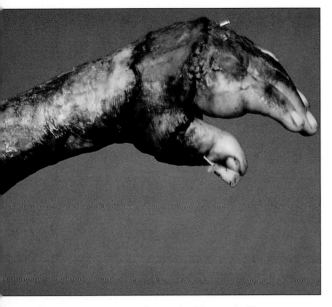

9.44 The same injury as shown in Figure 9.43 autografted and positioned with internal fixation. Note that all joints are in functional position.

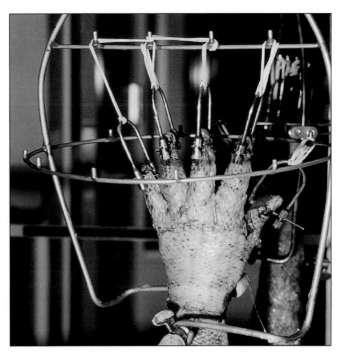

9.45 The banjo external fixator is useful in selected cases where deep structures are involved. Patients who have severe and extensive full thickness burns benefit from these procedures. The patient can actively mobilize all joints while the hand is maintained in proper position.

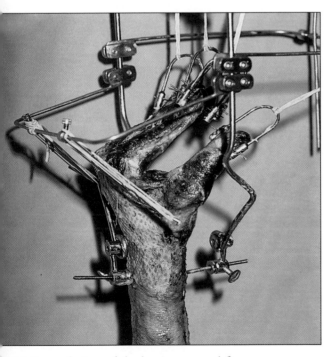

9.46 Lateral view of the banjo external fixator.

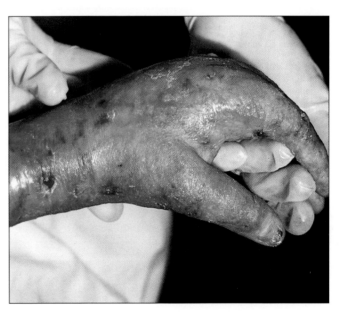

9.47 Good range of motion in all of the joints involved is achieved when all wounds are healed.

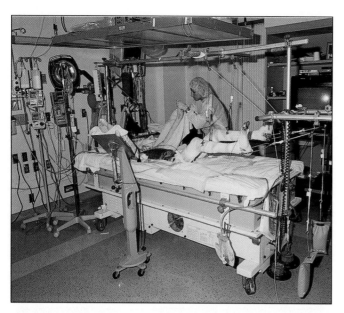

9.48 Skeletal traction is extremely useful in severe burns where there is paucity of donor sites and involvement of lower and upper limbs. A special frame attached to the bed is required for this technique.

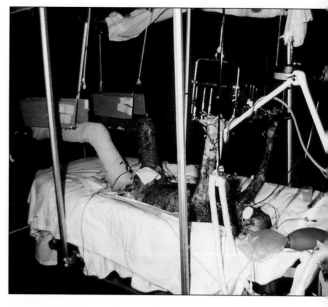

9.49 Complete active and passive range of motion exercises can be applied to all joints while in skeletal traction. Axillary and hip joints, however, are at risk for developing contractures, so special attention needs to be taken to increase passive and active exercising of these joints.

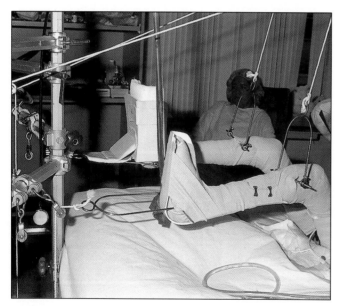

9.50 Positioning and dressing changes are more convenient for patients with severe burns who are treated with skeletal traction compared to those treated without. The forefoot also needs special attention in order to avoid plantar contractures.

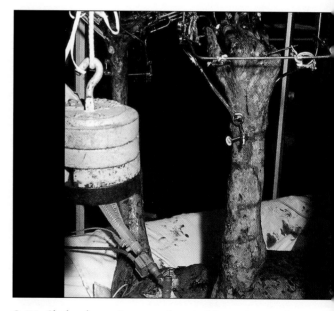

9.51 Skeletal traction may be used in patients whose wounds are closed with cultured epithelial autografts.

PRESSURE FOR SCAR MANAGEMENT

Options for pressure therapy in scar management
• Ace wraps
• Coban
• Tubigrip
• Interim garment
• Customized garment/Jobst
• Silicone inserts
• Silicone gels
• Face masks

.52 There are various ways to apply local pressure to
urn scars. Pressure therapy helps to reduce edema,
iminishes discomfort and itching problems, and helps in
car maturation.

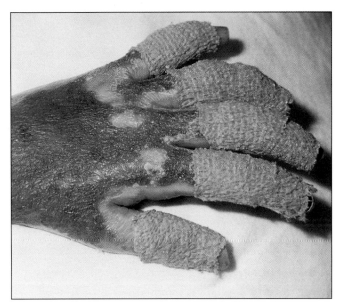

9.53 Coban bandages may be used to apply gentle
pressure to acral areas. Coban is useful during acute
recovery as interim measure for pressure therapy prior to
manufacture of Jobst garments.

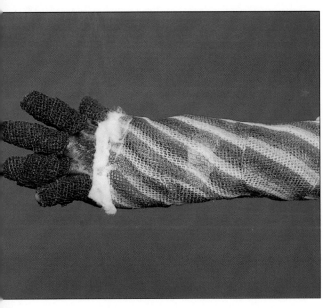

.54 Upper extremity treated with Coban. This kind of
pressure therapy is well tolerated by pediatric patients.

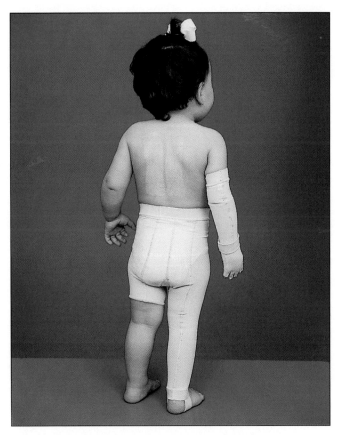

9.55 Customized pressure garments (Jobst) can be
tailored to the patient's needs, so that other areas may be
left uncovered.

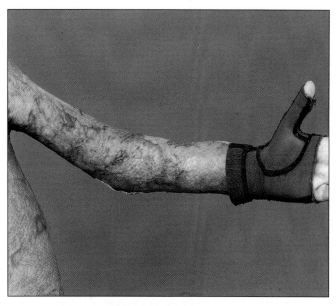

9.56 Jobst glove for burn scars to the hand. It is very important to explain the nature of burn scars to the patient and the positive effects that different pressure therapy devices may have on such injuries.

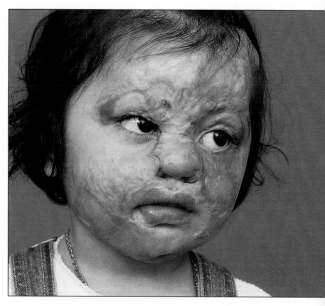

9.57 Burn scars to the face in a 2-year-old patient.

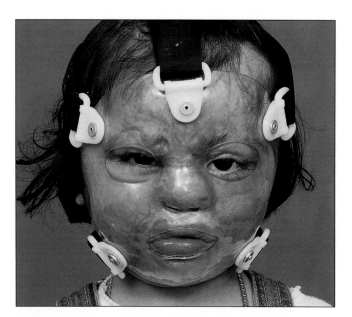

9.58 Facial scars treated with a U-vex mask. Some patients tolerate this transparent mask better than the moulage elastomer mask. Pressure applied to the scars is similar (same patient as shown in Figure 9.57).

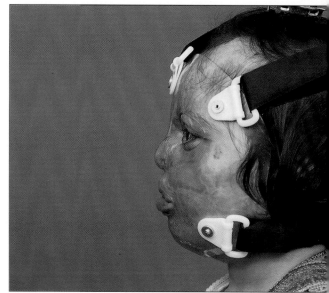

9.59 Lateral view of the patient shown in Figure 9.57.

PROSTHETIC AND ORTHOTIC INTERVENTION

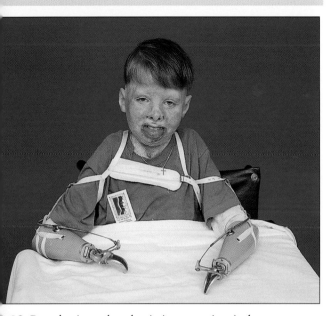

9.60 Prosthetic and orthotic intervention in burn patients is also part of the acute care plan. If prostheses are required, any sockets involved must be adjusted for permanent use at an early stage of hospital treatment, and patients should be provided with temporary devices early on so that rehabilitation programs can be started as soon as possible.

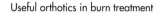

Useful orthotics in burn treatment
• Shoe inserts
• Orthopedic shoes
• Metatarsal bars with shank
• Ankle–foot orthoses
• Knee–ankle–foot orthoses
• Hip–knee–ankle–foot orthoses

9.61 Prosthetic and orthotic intervention is also an essential part of the work of the rehabilitation team in burn centers.

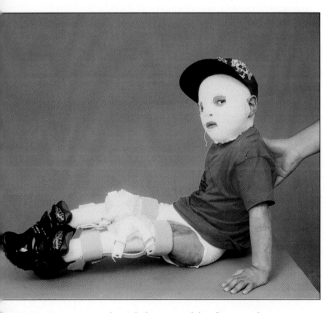

9.62 Patient treated with knee–ankle–foot orthoses, orthopedic shoes, and moulage elastomer facial mask.

CHAPTER 10

ESSENTIALS OF BURN RECONSTRUCTION

Juan P. Barret, MD and Peter Dziewulski, FRCS, FRCS(Plast)

GENERAL PRINCIPLES OF BURN RECONSTRUCTION

Essentials of burn reconstruction

- Reconstruction starts at the time of initial injury
- All members of a burn team should participate in the overall planning of reconstruction
- Psychologic support, splinting, exercises, and pressure garments all affect the surgical result
- Patients must also be included in this planning and understand the surgical objectives
- Dreams of miracles too often overshadow realistic goals and expectations
- The physician must encourage patients through the difficult acute period and also during reconstruction, but false expectations must be avoided
- Preoperative discussion minimizes postsurgical depression by improving patient acceptance

---

10.1 The reconstruction of the injury of the burn patient is a complex and lengthy process that usually starts at the time of the initial injury and often lasts from years to a lifetime. An excellent patient–surgeon relationship is essential.

Useful techniques during the acute phase

- Minimize edema
- Prevent conversion to full thickness injuries
- Start active and passive mobilization and ambulation as soon as possible
- Elevate and splint all limbs and joints
- Use darts with escharotomies to prevent linear contractures across joints
- Place graft seams that follow skin lines
- Place grafts on joints transversely
- Use sheet grafts whenever possible
- Avoid widely expanded mesh grafts
- Excise and autograft all wounds that do not heal within 3 weeks of injury
- Use cosmetic units when necessary
- Start rehabilitation and pressure therapy as soon as possible

---

10.2 Many techniques are very important during the acute phase to minimize late reconstructive problems. Attention to detail and early involvement of the reconstructive surgeon in the acute care of the injury is of paramount importance.

Timing of reconstruction	
Early reconstruction (scars immature)	Progressive deformity Progressive functional deficit
Late reconstruction	Progressive functional deficits not present Deformities stable and scars mature

---

10.3 Timing of the reconstruction is essential. It is always better to operate on mature scars, although when important functional deficits or involvement of important structures are present, early reconstruction operations are beneficial.

Priorities for reconstruction

- First priority must always remain the prevention of deformity
- Second priority is reconstruction of active function
- Final priority is restoration of passive function

10.4 Reconstruction proceeds stepwise, with priorities given to certain anatomic areas. What should be reconstructed becomes clear when one considers a patient as a whole.

Nonsurgical approach to burn reconstruction

• Compression
    Elasticized bandages (ace wraps)
    Tubular compression bandages (tubigrip)
    Ready-made garments and custom-fitted garments (Jobst)
• Silicone gel sheets
• Steroids
• Masks
• Splints

10.5 The same techniques that are useful in the acute phase are useful during the reconstructive phase in order to prevent and treat burn deformity.

The burn scar – problems encountered in burn reconstruction
• Hypertrophy • Atrophy • Keloids • Hyper- and hypopigmentation • Hyperkeratosis • Chronic open wounds • Contractures and tissue deficits • Anatomic deformities • Contour deformities • Partial and total amputation and absence of anatomic parts

10.6 Burn sequelae present a wide range of different problems that demand great experience from the plastic surgeon.

PROBLEMS ENCOUNTERED IN BURN RECONSTRUCTION

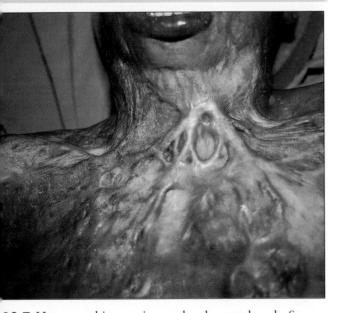

10.7 Hypertrophic scarring to the chest and neck. Scars that extend from the lower lip to the anterior chest result in severe functional deficit.

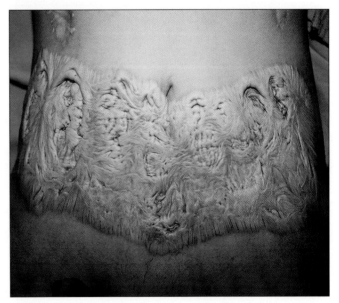

10.8 Hypertrophic scars to an abdominal donor site. Skin grafts harvested too deeply may result in such an outcome.

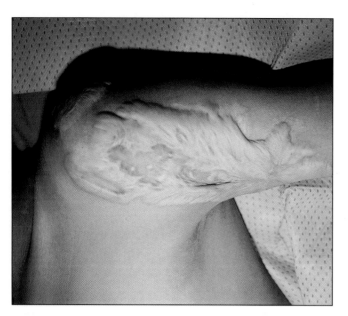

10.9 Hypertrophic scars from a healed deep second-degree burn. Burns that require more than 3 weeks to heal have a more favorable cosmetic and functional outcome if they are grafted during the acute period.

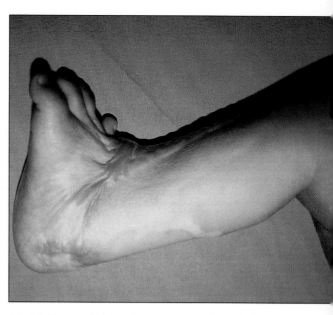

10.10 Burns that heal spontaneously and that are neglected may result in severe deformities that are very debilitating.

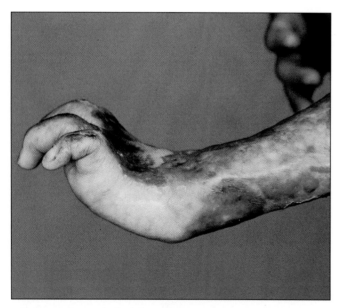

10.11 Intensive rehabilitation programs are extremely important during the acute phase and during reconstruction. They prevent severe deformity, which, when present, requires complex reconstructive operations.

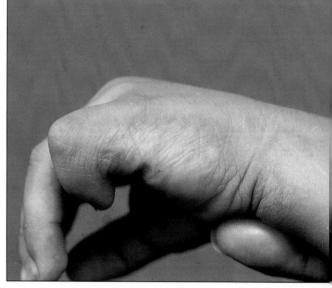

10.12 Severe contracture to the fifth finger. Reconstruction is usually necessary in this anatomic location. A 25% chance of recurrence should be expected with this particular deformity.

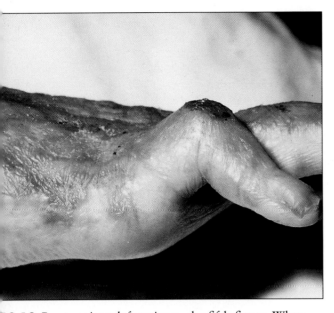

10.13 Boutonniere deformity to the fifth finger. When this deformity occurs and there is attenuation or disruption of the central extensor slit, reconstruction of the extensor mechanism is needed. If lateral bands are put under too much tension at the time of reconstruction, they may prevent flexion of the distal phalanx.

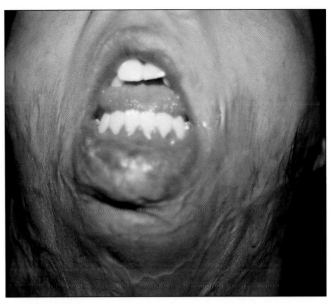

10.14 Severe lower lip ectropion. When reconstruction is needed, partial vermilionectomy or wedge excision may be required to maintain the tension of the muscle.

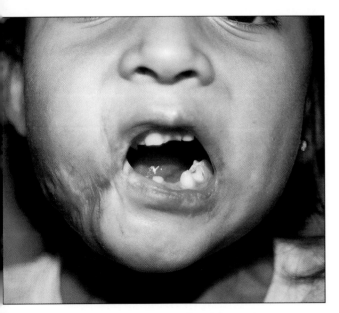

10.15 Burn scar contracture to the right oral commissure and cheek. Right oral commissuroplasty with mucosal flaps is often necessary. Tongue flaps are reserved for severe cases. If a tongue flap employed, it should not be visible at the lip to maintain normal cosmetic appearance.

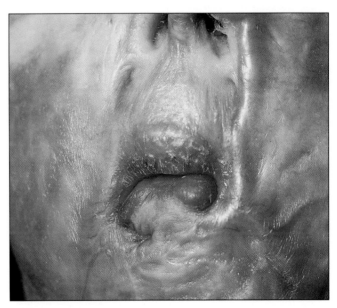

10.16 Severe microstomia in a 4-year-old patient. When circular scars exist around the mouth area, immediate prevention with mouth spreaders is mandatory.

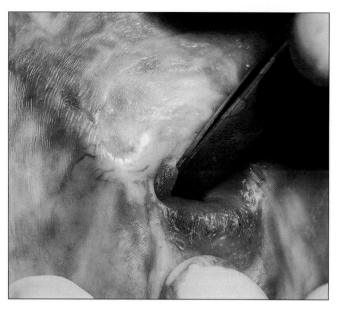

10.17 Close-up view of the patient shown in Figure 10.16. In these situations, early reconstruction is necessary, since the deformity interferes with feeding and speech.

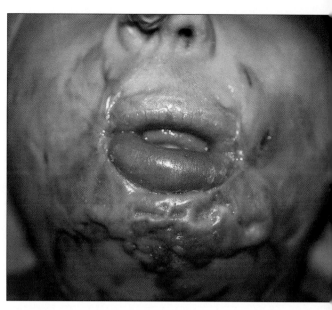

10.18 Mild microstomia and lower lip ectropion. Note that scars are still immature.

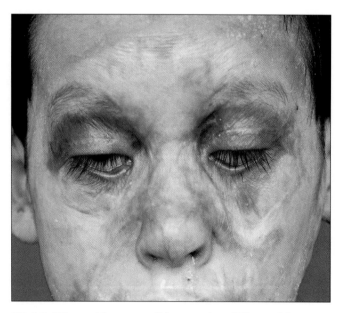

10.19 Bilateral lower eyelid ectropion. When addressing contractures to the eyelids and lips, it is important to ascertain whether they are caused by scars that affect the structure of the anatomic area (intrinsic) or whether they are caused by forces transmitted from other adjacent areas affected by scar contractures (extrinsic).

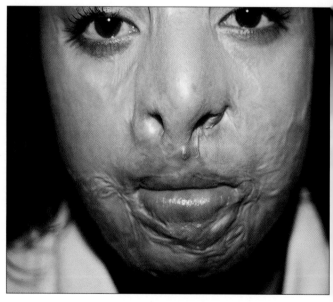

10.20 Burn scars to the upper and lower lips and to the tip of the nose. When contemplating nose reconstruction, it is essential to reconstruct first the upper lip, and then to concentrate on the nose.

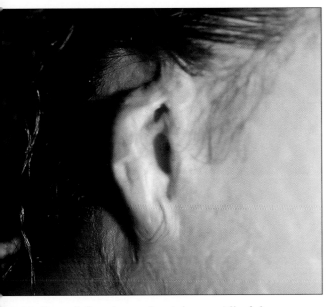

10.21 Burn deformity to the right ear. All of the cartilage is usually present, but is folded by the contracture. Release of the contracture and coverage with available tissue is sufficient to give a natural appearance.

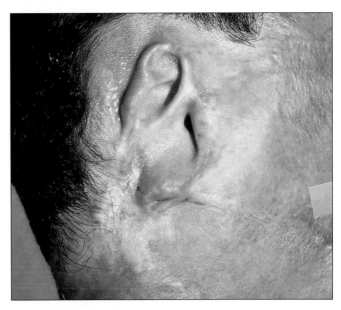

10.22 When total absence of the helical rim is encountered, ear reconstruction with rib cartilage graft with or without a temporalis fascia flap is normally necessary.

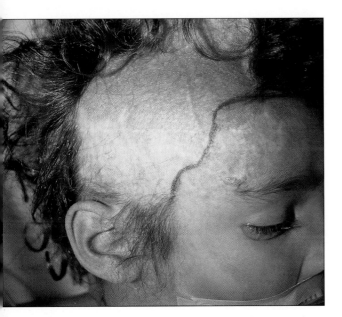

10.23 Burn scar alopecia. This sequela can be treated effectively with tissue expansion.

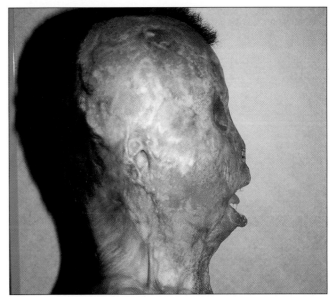

10.24 Severe burn deformity to the head and neck. This patient presents with burn scar alopecia, partial amputation of the nose, right face deformity, lower lip ectropion, enucleation of the right eye, and neck contracture. A comprehensive team approach is necessary in these situations to render the best outcome.

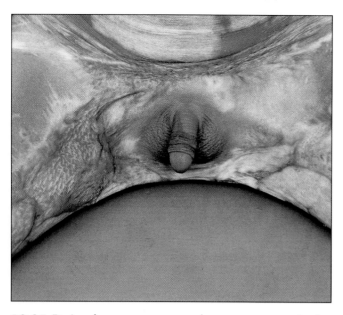

10.25 Perineal contractures are also very common in the pediatric population.

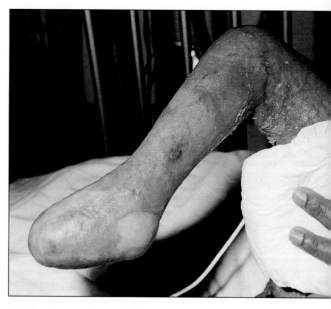

10.26 Severe burn deformity to the lower extremities with popliteal contractures and equinovarus deformity.

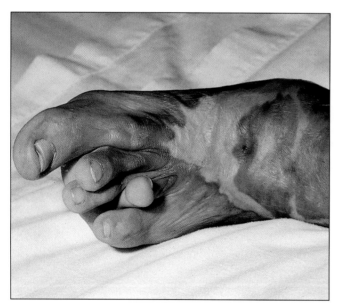

10.27 Hyper- and hypopigmentation are also burn sequelae that accompany burn contractures, hypertrophy and healing of second-degree burns and donor sites.

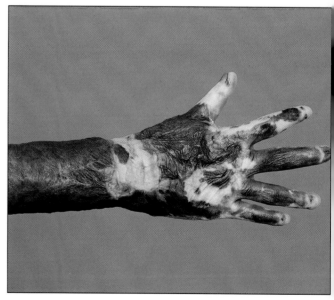

10.28 Changes in pigmentation can sometimes be more debilitating for patients than burn scarring.

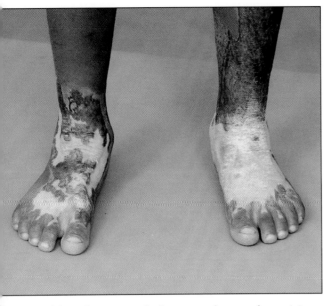

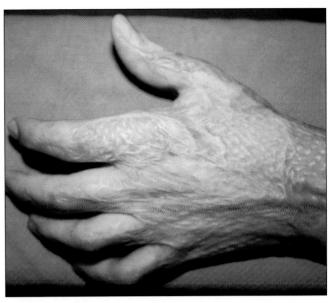

10.29 Although some techniques, such as early excision and grafting, pressure therapy, and dermal substitutes, have been proved effective to some extent in controlling scarring, there is currently no technique to control changes in pigmentation.

10.30 Mesh grafts should be avoided in small burns and reserved for hidden areas in severe burns. The mesh pattern leaves an ugly scar that is permanent.

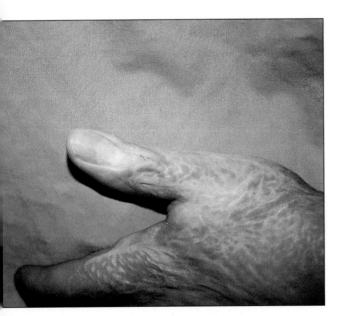

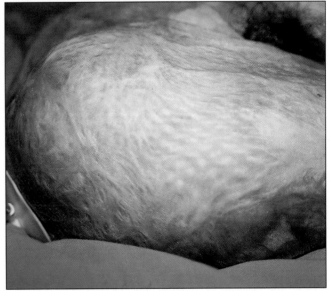

10.31 Close-up view of the same patient as shown in Figure 10.30 showing the mesh pattern and a nail deformity. Flaps and skin grafts are very useful for nail reconstruction.

10.32 Mesh pattern to the upper extremity. Sheet grafts should be used whenever possible in burn surgery. Even the 1:1 mesh leaves scars to the skin, so sheet grafts without cuts to ensure drainage should be used. In extensive burns, dermal substitutes are an excellent option to improve the outcome.

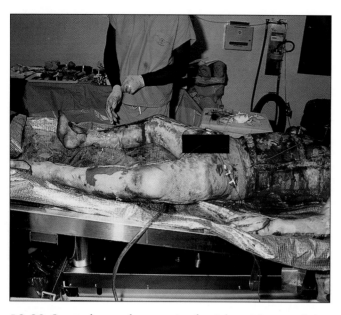

10.33 Severe burns that require fascial excision result in contour deformities that are very difficult to reconstruct.

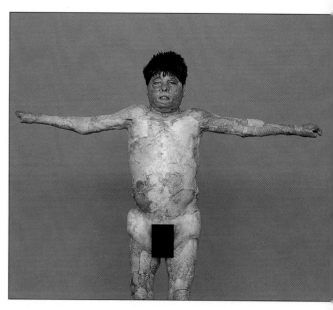

10.34 The same patient as shown in Figure 10.33 after treatment. Note the severe contour deformities to the abdomen and lower extremities.

OVERVIEW OF BURN RECONSTRUCTION

Techniques for burn reconstruction

- Excision and direct closure
- Scar realignment (Z-plasties and modifications)
- Split thickness skin grafts
- Full thickness skin grafts
- Composite grafts
- Cartilage and bone grafts
- Cutaneous or random pattern flaps
- Axial or arterial pattern flap
- Myocutaneous and osteomyocutaneous flaps
- Free flaps
- Expanded skin

10.35 All the techniques that are available for general plastic surgery patients are applicable to burn patients. Excellent pre-, intra-, and postoperative care and careful selection of the donor site and evaluation of the needs of the patient ensure the best outcome.

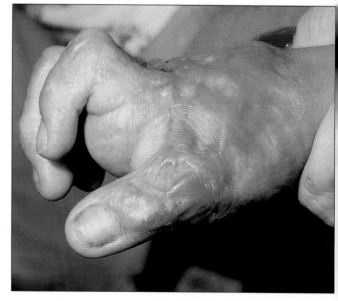

10.36 Burn scar deformity to the hand (typical claw appearance).

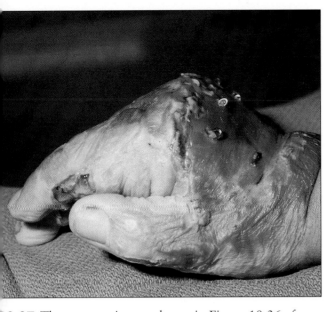

10.37 The same patient as shown in Figure 10.36 after burn scar release and split thickness autografting. When tissue deficit exists and tendons are protected by paratenon or subcutaneous tissue, skin autografts with or without k-wires are a good reconstructive option.

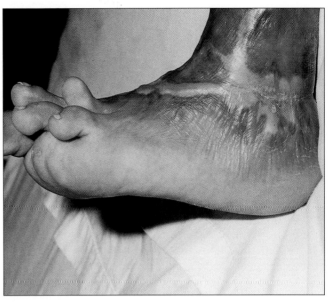

10.38 Burn scar deformity to the dorsum of the foot. Note the extension of the deformity to the toes.

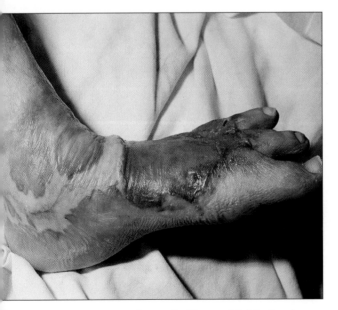

10.39 Same patient as shown in Figure 10.38 after burn scar contracture release and skin autografting.

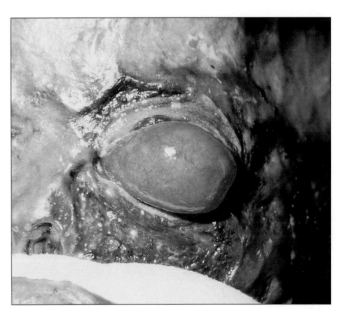

10.40 Severe contracture to the upper and lower eyelids with eversion of the conjunctiva.

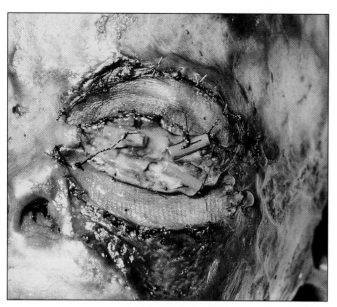

10.41 The same patient as shown in Figure 10.40 after upper and lower eyelid release. In normal circumstances, only one eyelid should be operated on at a time, to allow overcorrection of the deformity. All muscles and structures must be handled with extreme care to avoid further injury.

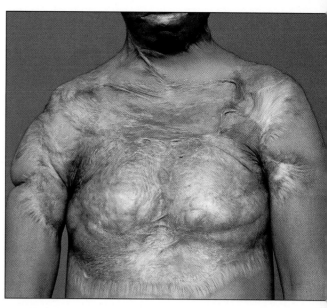

10.42 Burn scar contracture with breast deformity. Burns to the breast provoke severe deformities, especially in girls who are still in the process of development.

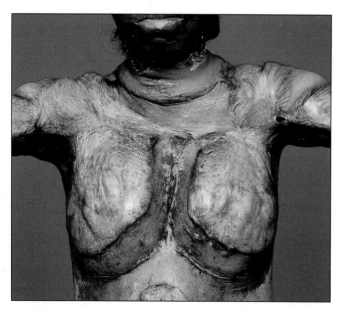

10.43 The inverted-T release is very helpful for this kind of reconstruction. Silicone inserts and sternal straps help to improve scarring and maintain shape.

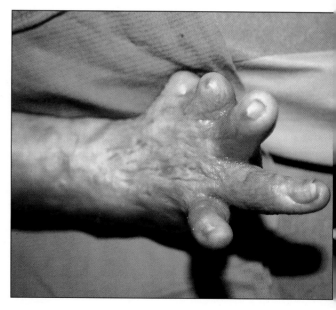

10.44 Severe burn contractures to the hand with partial amputation are a challenge to the burn team. As well as rehabilitation, complex operations are often necessary.

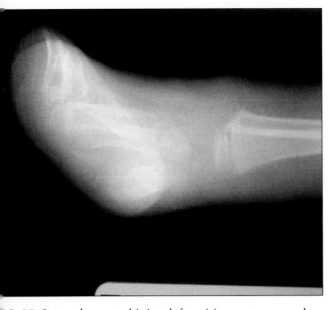

10.45 Severe bone and joint deformities accompany the burn sequelae shown in Figure 10.44.

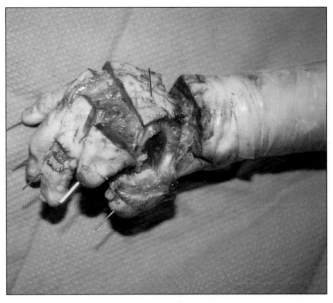

10.46 The first stage of reconstruction involves release of the burn scar, open capsulotomies, tenolysis, and skin coverage. In subsequent stages, metacarpal transfers or toe-to-thumb transfers may be attempted.

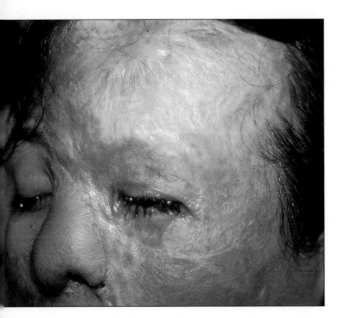

10.47 Burn scar deformity to the face and absence of the eyebrow.

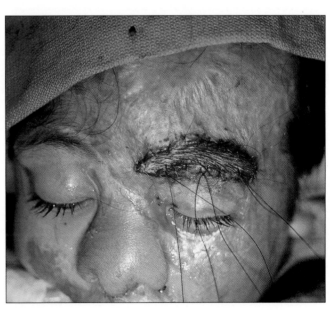

10.48 Reconstruction with composite graft from the scalp.

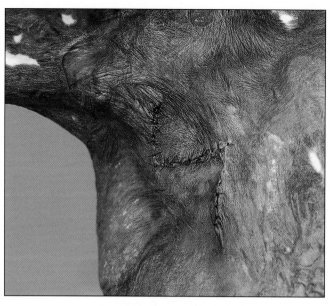

10.49 The Z-plasty technique. It is very helpful to break linear contractures in burn patients. If the flaps are well designed and enough subcutaneous tissue is included in them, preserving the damaged dermal plexus, then flaps that include burn scar tissue can be safely raised.

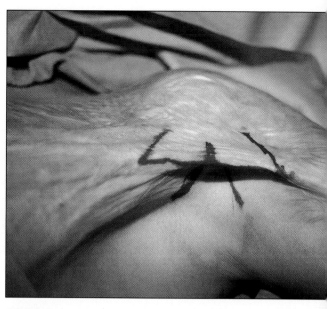

10.50 Burn scar contracture to the anterior axillary line. Note that five-limb Z-plasty or trident flaps have been designed.

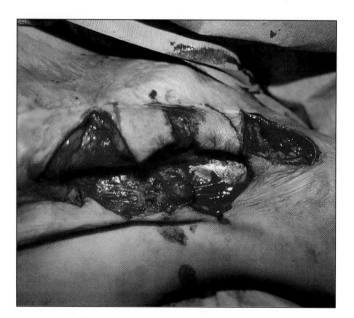

10.51 All flaps have been raised and hemostasis achieved. Hemostasis is imperative, because even a small hematoma may destroy such delicate flaps.

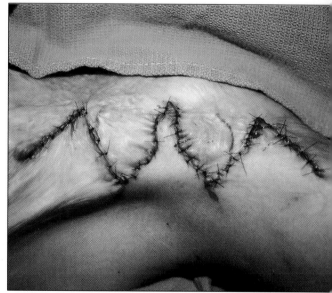

10.52 Final result with the flaps transposed.

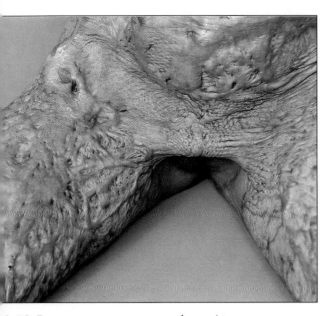

0.53 Burn scar contracture to the perineum.

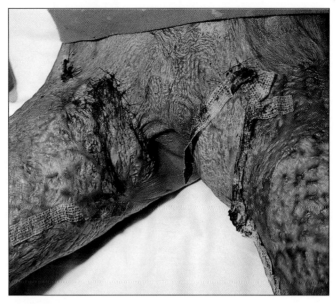

10.54 Reconstruction with bilateral internal fasciocutaneous flaps. Inclusion of the fascia in the flaps increases their viability. Good knowledge of the local and regional anatomy is necessary for correct design and performance of these flaps.

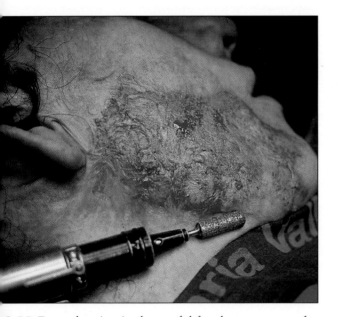

0.55 Dermabrasion is also useful for the treatment of burn sequelae. It can be used in region with scar irregularities to smooth the appearance of the anatomic region. Other useful techniques include chemical peels and depigmenting agents.

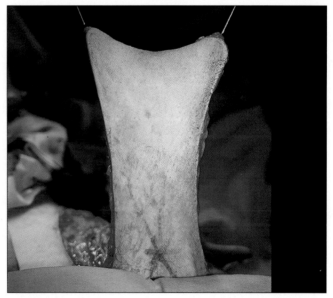

10.56 Direct axial cutaneous flaps, such as groin flaps, can be used pedicled or as free flaps to resurface or supply tissue to areas with skin and subcutaneous deficit. If inclusion of other tissues is required, this can be allowed for in the design of the flap. Groin flaps are very useful to reconstruct the dorsum of the hand when tendon support is required.

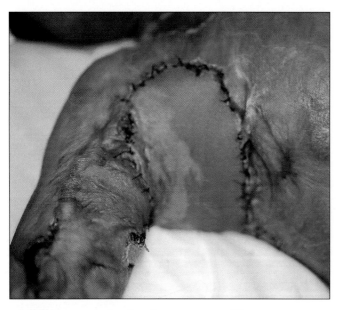

10.57 Parascapular flap for a severe axillary contracture. If a flap can be used for burn reconstruction, contracture is unlikely to recur. Moreover, the patient can start rehabilitation earlier than with skin grafts. It must be noted that neck and axillary contractures cannot be treated simultaneously, because positioning in bed cannot accommodate both of these sites.

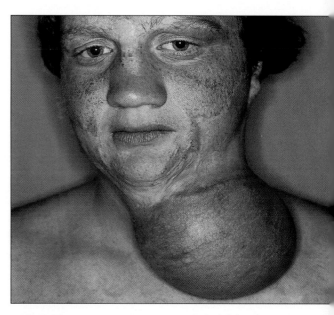

10.58 Tissue expansion is very helpful for face resurfacing. If neck tissue is available, neck tissue expanders can be placed and over-expanded to achieve the best outcome.

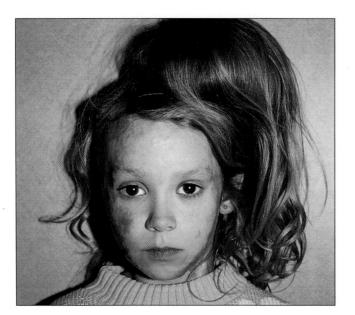

10.59 Tissue expansion is also very successful in the treatment of burn scar alopecia. Nose reconstruction and breast reconstruction are other areas where tissue expansion is useful in burn reconstruction.

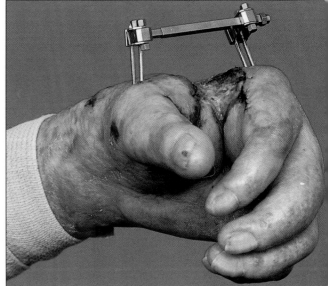

10.60 In severe contractures, where maintaining space and stretching soft tissues is important, external fixation is a good option.

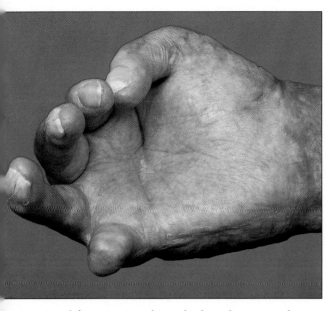

10.61 Good function is achieved when the external fixation device is removed.

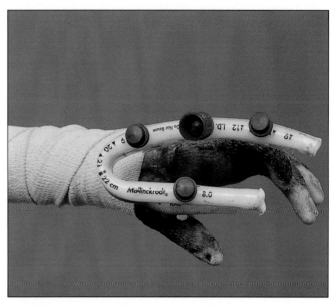

10.62 Methylmethacrylate external fixators can also be used for maintenance of space and stretching soft tissues. They maintain the hand in proper functional position with k-wires.

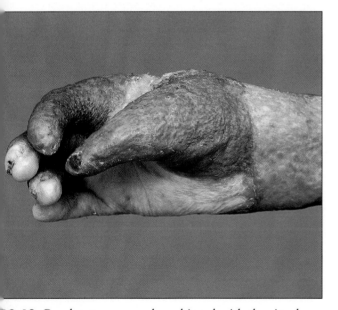

10.63 Good outcome can be achieved with the simple method of fixation shown in Figure 10.62.

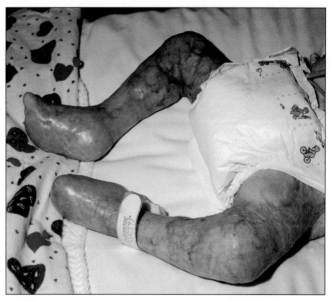

10.64 Severe contractures to the lower and upper extremities with extensive retraction of soft tissues and muscle and joint structures, can also be treated using external fixators.

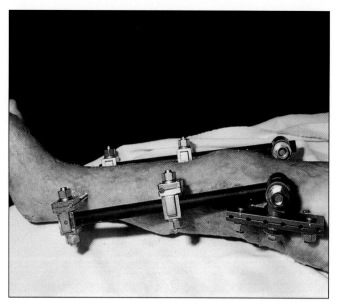

10.65 Same patient as shown in Figure 10.64 after burn scar contracture release, autografting, and fixation with AO system.

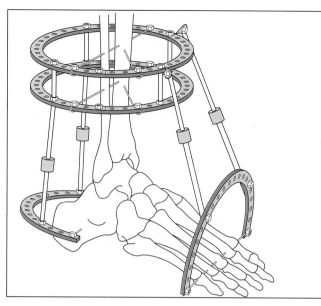

10.66 The Ilizarov technique is very helpful for the treatment of equinovarus deformity. In knee and elbow contractures, mobilization is performed over a fixed period. Good motion can be achieved even in severe ankylosis.

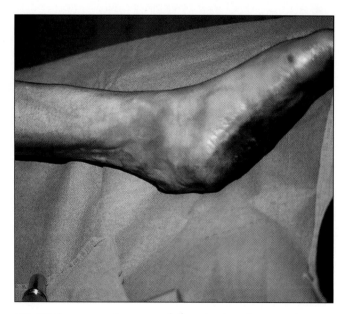

10.67 Severe equinovarus deformity in a burn patient.

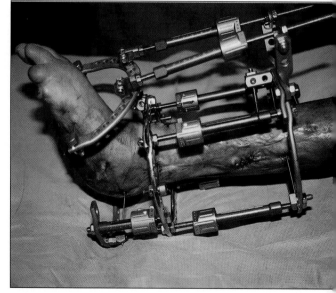

10.68 The complete Ilizarov framework in place. Over a period of time the framework is stretched by turning specific screws, achieving complete correction of the deformity.

CHAPTER 11
NOMOGRAMS AND USEFUL INFORMATION

Marc G. Jeschke, MD

Lund and Browder chart

Age	0–1	1–4	5–9	10–14	15
A – 1/2 of head	9 1/2%	8 1/2%	6 1/2%	5 1/2%	4 1/2%
B – 1/2 of one thigh	2 3/4%	3 1/4%	4%	4 1/4%	4 1/2%
C – 1/2 of one leg	2 1/2%	2 1/2%	2 3/4%	3%	3 1/2%

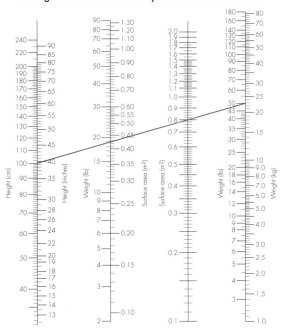

11.1 Lund and Browder chart. An estimation of burn size and depth supports the determination of severity, prognosis, and disposition of a thermally injured patient. Burn size directly affects fluid resuscitation, nutritional support, and surgical interventions. To determine the accurate size in burn patients the Lund and Browder chart is used clinically. (Adapted from Herndon DN, ed. Total Burn Care, WB Saunders, 1996)

Nomogram to estimate the body surface area for adults

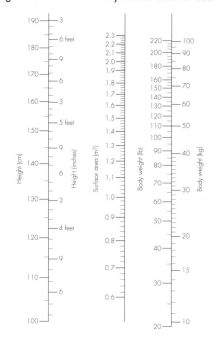

11.2 Nomogram to estimate the body surface area for adults. Body surface area estimation represents a guide to fluid resuscitation and nutritional support. Body surface area can be calculated from height and weight using standard nomograms. (UTMB admission form, Galveston, Texas)

Nomogram to estimate the body surface area for children

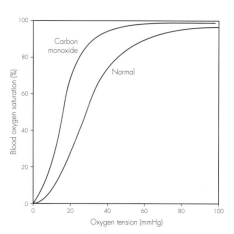

11.3 Nomogram to estimate the body surface area for children. The example depicted is for a child 100cm in height and 23kg in weight, resulting in 0.8m² body surface area. (Adapted from Eichelberger MR, ed "pediatric trauma: prevention, acute care and rehabilitation", Mosby year book St. Louis, 1993)

11.4 Carbon monoxide toxicity remains one of the most frequent immediate causes of deaths following inhalation injury. Carbon monoxide toxicity must be suspected in every fire victim and must be treated. The half-life of carbon monoxide in room air is 250min and in patients breathing 100% oxygen, 40–60min. The oxygen–hemoglobin dissociation curve relates oxygen tension, oxygen saturation, and oxygen content. If the curve shifts to the right, hemoglobin has less affinity for oxygen and releases oxygen more rapidly. Carbon monoxide causes a left-shift, which means that hemoglobin binds oxygen more vigorously and inhibits oxygen release to the tissue. (Adapted from Strongin S, et al. In "pulmonary disorders in the burn patient", acute management of de burned patient, WB Saunders Philadelphia, 1990)

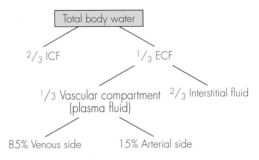

11.5 Fluid composition of the body. In a normal human, about 60% of the total body weight is water (e.g. 42l in a 70kg man). Approximately two-thirds of this fluid resides inside cells and is called intracellular fluid (ICF). One-third of the water is extracellular [the extracellular fluid (ECF)]. The ECF can be further divided into the interstitial fluid compartment (fluid between cells), which constitutes two-thirds of the ECF, and the vascular compartment (plasma fluid), which contains about one-third of the ECF. Of the vascular fluid 85% resides in the venous system and 15% in the arterial system.

Normal water and electrolyte balance for children and adults		
	Adults	**Children**
Water	30–50ml/kg body weight/day	100ml – [3 × age (years)]ml × kg body weight
Electrolyte		
Sodium	50–90mmol/l per day	3mmol/l per kg body weight/day
Potassium	40–90mmol/l per day	3mmol/l per kg body weight/day
Chloride	50–90mmol/l per day	2–3mmol/l per kg body weight/day
Magnesium	10–25mmol/l per day	1–2mmol/l per kg body weight/day

11.6 Normal water and electrolyte requirements for children and adults. The normal adult ingests 2–2.5l/day and loses 0.8–1.5l through urine, 0.25l through stool, and 0.6–0.9l through insensible loss. In children the amount is dependent on age and body weight.

APPENDIX

Acticoat: Westaim Biomedical Inc.
1 Hampton Rd, Suite 302
Exeter, N.H. 03833

Adaptic/Xeroform: Johnson & Johnson Medical Inc.
2500 E. Arbrook Blvd.
Arlington, Texas 76104

Biobrane: Bertek Pharmaceuticals Inc.
3711 Collins Ferry Rd.
Morgantown, WV 26504

Mepitel: Molnlycke Healthcare
500 Baldwin Tower
Eddystone, PA 19022

Dermagraft: Informagen Inc.
375 Little Bay Rd.
Newington, NH 03801

Opsite: Smith and Nephew Wound Care
11775 Starkey
Largo, FL 33779

INDEX

inal cord injuries 32
ine, cause of deformities to 138
linting
custom-made 148
general principles 146
fingers 147
thumb 147
ukulele 148
uninjured areas and 147
lit autografts 84
uamous cell carcinoma 129
aged surgical wound closure 84
aphylococcus aureus 115–16
aphylococcus spp. 114
arling equation 48
bclavian line 39, 42
bcutaneous vascular plexus, thromboses 5
bglottic carbon clot 54
bglottic tracheal hemorrhagic spots 57
bmucosal injury 50
bstance abuse patients 12
cralfate 133
ulfamylon cream/solution 78
rgical techniques 84
wab–Ganz catheter 40
weat glands 2, 3, 4
wis and swallow' 116
ystemic effects of burn wound 9
ystemic inflammatory response syndrome (SIRS) 10

angential excision 84
annic acid 76
attoo, long-term 17
emperature
maintenance 88
core, monitoring 38
probes 38
hermal brain injury 21
hird-degree burn (full thickness burn) 5–6, 11, 21–2
horacostomy, tube 132
hrombophlebitis 120, 131
risk of 39
hrombosis
risk of 39
septic 131
humb, deformity 141
issue expansion 91, 170
ongue flaps 159
otal burn wound excision 84
ourniquets, tangential excision under 96–7
oxic epidermal necrolysis 24–5
oxic smoke compounds 48
rachea, erythema 55
racheal-bronchial hemorrhage 57

tracheal cast 56, 58
tracheal esophageal fistula 64
tracheal hemorrhage 56
tracheal malacia 65
tracheal scarring 64
tracheal stenosis 63–4
tracheobronchitis, necrotizing 50, 55, 131
tracheostomy 63, 87
traction
on eschar 93
skeletal 91, 150
transfer to burn center 40
transportation to burn center 40–1
trauma
patients 28
road accident 30–1
trident flap 168
TRNSCYTE 107
tube fixation 85
tubular necrosis, acute 134

ukulele splint 148
University of Texas Medical branch, Galveston 43
urine, alkalinization 16
U-vex mask 152

vascular compartment 175
vasodilatation 71, 72
vasopressors 130
vermilionectomy 159
volumetric diffusive respiration ventilator 68
volumetric diffusive respiration wave form 68

water balance 175
Watson dermatome 90, 93
wedge excision 159
wound care 75
wound closure
in non-life-threatening burns 84
techniques 85
wound healing
considerations 70
principles 70
spontaneous 74, 158
wounds that benefit from excision and grafting 84
wrist, physical deformities 140

Zimmer dermatome 91, 98
zinc, molten 14
zone of hyperemia 7
zone of necrosis 7
zone of stasis 7, 8, 18
Z-plasty 168